THE
BEAUTIFUL
PEOPLE'S
DIET BOOK

THE
BEAUTIFUL
PEOPLE'S
DIET BOOK

LUCIANA AVEDON

and Jeanne Molli

Saturday Review Press / E. P. Dutton & Co., Inc.

New York

Published simultaneously in Canada by
Doubleday Canada Ltd., Toronto.

Library of Congress catalog card number: 72–88646
ISBN 0–8415–0280–3

PRINTED IN THE UNITED STATES OF AMERICA
Design by Tere LoPrete

Contents

Introduction

There are the cheetahs of this world, and the hippopotami. Much to my chagrin, I was built for the herd—one year of negligence and you would find me by the riverbank, shifting my bulk in a vast hippopotamus sprawl.

I love to eat; I always have. My bones are big and I am tall enough to long for other times when one dressed in flowing robes and carried fat with majesty and pride. To be lean was then to be mean or, worse, to be poor.

Instead I live in contemporary Rome, where, as in any big city nowadays, you have to be thin to be chic. You have to be thin to feel still attractive and vital once past thirty, and if such matters—I can hear you protest—are not your concern, the alternatives are nil. Your doctor will preach that you have to be thin for your health.

In *The Beautiful People's Beauty Book,* I touched on the disciplines of exercise and simple eating. I did not write at length on these because it seemed so obvious that they were basic habits to acquire like remembering to brush your teeth, say please, and take the garbage out. Unfortunately, for most of us, staying in shape is not a basic habit. We do not grow up applying the rules every day, much less find ready examples to follow in the immediate family.

Yet the sooner you start, the easier it is to develop an appetite for exercise and curb the one for food. Maybe I was lucky (though I doubt it) to be such a mess in my teens—lucky to catch that hippo rump when my body was still young and sufficiently pliant to assume another form. My adolescence was thick, so much so I swore it would never happen again.

I am now thirty-eight and, at five feet seven, tip the scales at 127 pounds. Give or take five digits, I have stayed at this weight for almost fifteen years. No one would ever say I was skinny, but I dare them to find a pound I should lose.

I've had to learn it all the hard way, but I learned just the same, at first by making mistakes. Gradually I adopted an empirical, personal system. Now, if you ask me how many calories there are in a glass of wine, two ounces of green beans, or eight ounces of broiled steak, I cannot tell you unless I look it up. On the other hand, it is quite clear in my mind that reaching for a second apple is not the same as having two plates of spaghetti, and I act accordingly. At a certain point, one stops counting every calorie, just as one stops taking rides on the merry-go-round of miracle diets. Baby, you know what is good for you, and that is what you eat.

You still eat well. Long-term dieting has never meant, unless you like the stuff, that you sign on for a perpetual lunch of Nixonian cottage cheese (large-curd or not, with or without ketchup). It does mean that, once past adolescence, you refrain from such Humphrey specials as peanut butter, bologna, cheddar cheese, lettuce, and mayonnaise on toasted bread with lots of ketchup on the side.

If you are looking for the catechism on what is a calorie or what is a balanced diet (whose balance, I might ask?), this is not the book for you. Any number of other books, charts, and pamphlets can spell that out. Most probably you were taught the basic tenets in school, where unless the knowledge was applied, it went in one ear, out the other like calculus or the names of the kings of France.

(Just for the record, the catechism goes as follows:

Q. What is a calorie?
A. A calorie is a measure of energy chiefly obtained from food.
Q. How do calories affect weight?
A. If the body takes in more calories than it burns up in energy, the excess makes you fat.
Q. Are the foods highest in calories most nutritious?
A. Not necessarily. For example, the body needs protein, it can do without cake.
Q. What are the best foods from the point of view of slimness and nutrition?
A. The best foods for slimness are those that provide protein, vitamins, and minerals; fats and carbohydrates to be consumed in lesser quantities for balanced nutrition.)

The question, however, is not just getting the answers right, but also scoring at the table, where it counts. When I was last in Paris, I went backstage at the Crazy Horse Saloon to see what the strippers thought about dieting. The four girls I talked with, Bonita, Capsula Pop, Franca Torpedo, and Madlena, were all in their twenties, an age when one tends to take the body beautiful for granted. Not the strippers! None of them was on a diet and sometimes they nibbled or splurged, but, as it turned out, basically they all ate broiled meat, fish, salad, dairy products, and fruit. With that routine, plus exercise, who needs a diet? (One useful tip from the girls:

when you want to look great in the nude, cut down on liquid intake. It is all right to drink after the show; do it before and you look bloated. Do not overeat before or you feel heavy and your legs are not with you.)

One morning in Rome, when it was noticed that he put saccharin in his tea, Richard Burton spoke in the famous plural: "Neither of us has a real weight problem, so we don't take diets seriously. But they're fun to try. We've collected at least two hundred diet books."

For people who do have a problem, that must be par for the course. You collect books, and the books collect dust. Various diets are mentioned in this book, none of which I endorse, although as palliatives they seem to me as good as most. The opinions of various slimming experts and doctors are also listed. When it comes to specifics, they rarely agree, which is not surprising—diet is a controversial subject. Above all, I have quoted people who visibly have their weight under control. If I wanted tips on gardening, I would not ask someone whose plants looked unhappy. I would go to someone with a green thumb. In this case—how to stay thin—I have gone to the beautiful people who cannot afford to be fat. Neither can you. Can anyone?

THE
BEAUTIFUL
PEOPLE'S
DIET BOOK

1

Put a Buzzer on the Fridge

Put a buzzer on the fridge!

The idea hit me in Long Island as we set out to visit friends who lived just down a quiet road. We got into our rented car, turned the key in the ignition—and were buzzed out of our minds. The noise was loud, nonstop, and clearly designed to allow no exercise of judgment: it was a case of fasten your seat belts or else. All of us scrambled for buckles and straps.

That was when I thought of the refrigerator. If a buzzer can help reduce driving hazards, why can't it help reduce fat? You could rig the buzzer to go off every time the refrigerator is opened between meals. An alternate model would allow you to open sesame at any hour, but not more than ten times a day. Exceed the limit, and all hell breaks loose. As for staples, fatties would store them in locked cupboards and then, of course, deposit the keys inside the monitored icebox, a twentieth-century twist on the stingy medieval chatelaine who kept the keys to the larder on her person.

A fiendish idea? You bet. But in God we trust, not in you, says the car rental company as it buzzes you into fastening a seat belt. So why trust the careless, compulsive eater to stop the snacks that are digging his early grave? Of course, I know the buzzer would not work. Just as you learn to fool the buzzer in your car and still drive beltless, you would never tolerate a refrigerator that blasted you with bad vibrations—lit up and said tilt—every time you cheated. Still, something has to be done. These days it seems that the more storage space you have, the more you fill it, and, in consequence, the more you eat, because the stuff is there. Moreover, with the onslaught of processed foods, the quantity of goodies that can be stored is staggering—a manic eater's paradise. Until I married an American, I kept very little food around the house. Now you would think we lived in the wilderness where we risked being snowbound for weeks: the shelves are bulging. As long as *we* are not, I go along with this provident approach, but at the first signs of snackitis and sprawl, rest assured the cupboard will be bare.

Do not get me wrong. I am all for affluence, which is precisely why I hate to watch the affluent society gleefully opt for a Via Crucis to the fridge like lemmings swarming to the sea —in this case, a sea of fat. Because of modern techniques, food in Western countries is no longer in short supply; the need no longer prevails, when you bag a beast or the harvest is in, to glut because the winter may be long. As French diet specialist Colette Lefort remarks, "Moderation must take place of greediness in a world where everything is offered." This is not what has happened. For the moment, while the Third World still dies from starvation, the affluent society kills itself by overeating.

The dangers of obesity are public knowledge. For years, the warnings have been posted. Among the maladies linked to obesity, or aggravated by it, are: arteriosclerosis, arthritis, diabetes, digestive disorders, inflammation of the gallbladder, cirrhosis of the liver, heart disease, hernias of various sorts, high blood pressure, kidney disease, and varicose veins. Obesity also increases the chances of complications during pregnancy and delivery. Maybe the list should be stuck on the refrigerator.

"Overeating is worse than dope," says Mark D. Altschule, clinical professor of medicine at the Harvard Medical School, "because with dope the situation is clear. Dope is bad. But you can't say food is bad, so people eat and eat, and gradually they gain weight. Then, when they become too fat or are worried about becoming too fat, they start restricting their diet . . . usually in the wrong way." It has often been said that Americans are the most overfed and undernourished people on earth. One estimate is that fifty million Americans are either overweight or obese, a figure that Dr. Altschule finds conservative. (The difference between the two terms, which are often used interchangeably, is a matter of degree. For example, if you are supposed to weigh 110 pounds and you weigh 125, you are overweight. Tip the scales at 140, and you start to be obese.)

The high priestess of nutrition, Adelle Davis, has calculated that one out of three Americans suffers from excess weight. John Yudkin, professor of nutrition and dietetics, University of London, has estimated that less than a third of American men and women under thirty are overweight; on the other hand more than half the men and three-quarters of the women between the ages of forty-five and fifty-five have a weight problem. In other words, he stresses (in *This Slimming Business*) the importance of age and sex, rather than relying on overall statistics. In his opinion, the proportion of fat people in Britain is almost as high.

I do not think you have to resort to graphs and math to notice that you live in a world of bulges, spare tires, cellulite,

paunches—and diet crazes. Who has not tried some ineffectual, and possibly unhealthy, diet that promised miracles?
Who has not been bored by other people's weighty problems
and their inconstant resolves to reform? From sixteen to sixty,
most of us fight erratic skirmishes with the scales.

As for the risks involved not just in being overweight, but
also in making crash attempts at slimming, diet specialist Dr.
Neil Solomon has stated (in *The Truth About Weight Control*)
that more than 50 percent of the patients he interviewed at
the Johns Hopkins and Baltimore City hospitals had nutritional deficiencies. These were prevalent in an alarming degree among overweight patients who had been on a variety of
odd diets.

Somehow, I fear, one always thinks there must be a short
cut to slenderness, some drastic uphill climb one can manage
to pant through, because, after it's over, one will be home
free forever. Unfortunately, with food, this never seems to
work.

When I was growing up, there was one aunt in the family
who seemed to have spent her entire life on a diet. The diet
was never the same, although a recurrent favorite was the
one-of-a-kind system: one day of meat, one day of fruit, one
day of vegetables, and so on. She kept up with diets the way
other people keep up with the news; she was always on to the
latest thing. It finally dawned on me that maybe the diets
themselves were not so bad; it was what she did in between
that made her fat. She never talked about the interim periods
—she was probably too busy stuffing in the goodies.

As reported by *Time*, Dr. Alvan Feinstein of Yale Medical
School rates the success of weight-loss programs as "terrible,
much worse than in cancer." Furthermore, some doctors have
found that out of one hundred obese patients, only twelve
lose any substantial amount of weight during one year's treatment, and ten of these are likely to gain back their loss the
following year. These dismaying statistics were unfurled in

June, 1972, during a Washington medical meeting held in order to found the American Society of Bariatrics. Specializing in bariatrics means, in less distinguished terminology, dealing in fat. It was about time that the medical profession realized that fat doctors and fat research are of vital importance if preventive medicine is to have any real meaning.

So far there is no miracle formula for slimness. I have none. Nor do my friends, or for that matter, any of the various personalities and specialists who are quoted in this book. You read one qualified opinion, then another; you read fifty—and they all conflict. Also the infighting is ferocious, whether from laboratory conviction (but it still depends how the test is done!), intuitive feeling, or the hope of making a buck from the sale of some dubious nostrum.

Even the famous "balanced diet" composed of low-calorie doses of meat or meat substitutes, vegetables and fruit, dairy foods, and cereal products is not universally applauded. High-protein proponents question the need for carbohydrates; Swiss and English naturopaths have always played down the need for meat. Rome's Dr. Fulvio Rossi contends that "the well-balanced diet seems logical, but it isn't necessarily right. I had a patient who only ate potatoes; they were a sort of fixation. He was one of the healthiest men I've seen."

You have the three-meals-a-day-and-no-snacks school versus those who advise eating less at one time but eating more often. You have the big-breakfast boys versus the light-breakfast believers. Unless you have already gone to an early grave from saturated fats, additives, or pesticides, be assured (depending on your source) that white sugar, white bread, or salt will do you in. Vitamin pills are pushed; vitamin pills are scorned. Health foods will save your life; health foods are a racket. Line up your yin and yang, "Beware the Jabberwock, my son!" Beware the sanpaku. The only consensus seems to be that—whatever you eat and drink—than if you stoke in more calories than your body burns up, you get fat.

"People refuse to understand food," says New Yorker and beautiful former model Betsy Pickering (Mrs. Harilaos) Theodoracopulos. "Pick up any old calorie chart, and it is all quite clear. You see that lima beans have more calories than salad, and bacon more than lean meat, so if you like them, you have to allow for them. As for balanced diet, by now you learn about it along with your ABCs."

The trouble, I suppose, is that knowledge is not enough unless you act on it, and most of us balk when it comes to applying information that disagrees with us. This is true, of course, not only in nutrition but in almost any area from politics and love to finance and fashion. As Diana Vreeland, former editor-in-chief of *Vogue*, told me with her usual, quite devastating frankness, "You know, the shocking thing after thirty-four years in this business is that when you get out and look around, you realize that people haven't learned a thing—they just don't care."

With diet, the problem is more complex. People pretend to care—their fat is guilt-ridden—but they are torn between caring about staying in shape and loving to eat and drink. Food usually wins out because diet is equated with deprivation, something you resort to only in extremis. Instead, diet, as I see it, is a way of life (presumably a long one), because you prefer to eat what makes you feel good and also keeps you thin; you prefer it for aesthetic reasons and taste satisfaction as well as for health and a boost in energy. What is called for is consciousness raising, a food awareness that liberates rather than one that traps you in fat—a way with food that works for you versus the old emotional ties and eating habits that bog you down.

As glamorous French businesswoman Hélène Rochas says, "You have to make sensible eating pleasant. You won't believe in it otherwise."

I confess that my own initial interest in diet had nothing to do with health. (The health concern came later.) I wanted to be beautiful, and beautiful means, among other contemporary definitions, being slender. That was sufficient motivation for me.

It is not in my nature to be thin. If I just went ahead and ate any old way, within a year I would weigh a ton. In my case, the beauty drive was stronger than imagined hunger, and by my late twenties I had already found my second nature; I could eat pleasurably and still not put on weight.

"Anyone who tells me he doesn't diet is a liar," says Mrs. Winston (Ceezee) Guest. "Dieting is the most boring thing in the world, but if you want to have a good figure and look divine, you have to."

At the same time, Ceezee does not follow any arbitrary plan and would never go in for crash regimens. I myself never go on a diet, though I have my frugal days to compensate for occasional food orgies. Ask any number of lean, attractive people what they do, and their first reaction is always the same: "I don't do anything; I don't diet." Second reactions veer to apparent extremes: "I love to eat," or, "I'm just not all that interested in food." In practice, the extremes are reconciled. If you watch slender people eat—people still slender past thirty—you see that they demand both good food and little of it. They seem to have some built-in radar that keeps their eating in line with their ideal weight.

"I never hear women I know say 'I must go on a diet,' " Baroness Pauline de Rothschild remarks. "I hear them say sorrowfully, 'I've eaten too much.' I know people who cut down, but I don't know anybody who doesn't eat any old thing. It's a question of balance—if you like a double vodka, then you don't have a chocolate. You know that when you get overweight, you don't feel as well."

The beautiful people eat well and they are not fat. They respect their varying food traditions—American, English, French, Italian, you name it—and yet the needle on the scale barely oscillates. I do not call them saints or martyrs. I would certainly say they are motivated—looking their best is an important part of their lives. You might add that they also save the time and the money for sports, gym classes, masseurs, and rehaulings at beauty farms. But such assists alone cannot account for prolonged stabilizing of weight.

The beautiful people do not jump on and off the diet merry-go-round; in a sense, they have dieted all their lives and always will. By this I mean they have chosen, each one in a personal way, to eat thin and have learned to like it. There is really no other choice. Even if you start with a fifty-pound handicap, the process is the same. You transform what begins as an effort of will into an informed eating style that you would not trade for all the guzzling in the world.

Staying in shape, however you get there in the first place, cannot be done in spurts; it is a long-term race. And you have not won until you, too, protest that you never diet: "Dieting is such a bore!" That means that you no longer have to because your weight has been right for years. You have learned to eat.

2

How Do They Always Look So Good?

"I like to eat, I really do," says Aileen Mehle (society columnist Suzy), "but I know how much I should weigh, and the minute I go five pounds over, I cut back to 1,000 calories a day."

"I keep my weight fluctuation within two pounds. It's bad for the face when you go up and down," says California socialite Betsy (Mrs. Alfred) Bloomingdale. "Beyond two pounds, I eat half of everything until I'm back to normal."

I kept hearing the same words in London, Los Angeles, New York, Paris, and Rome. All those I talked to about staying in shape replied that their weight has not changed in years, because the minute it shoots up, they shoot it down. This is what I call the five-pound limit. I believe in it, and though I have scales in the house, I do not need them to tell me when the limit has been reached. I can feel it with or without my clothes on, and by now I am so conditioned that when I feel heavy I am not hungry. I automatically eat "light" until I am lean again.

I have also never needed a chart to tell me how much I should weigh, nor does anyone really. You see yourself and you know. As Hélène Rochas states, "You must have a mean mirror in the house. A flattering one won't do at all."

The five-pound limit on weight increase is stricter than the allowance given by life insurance companies. Led by the Metropolitan Life Insurance Company, they were pioneers in tabulating both average and desirable weight according to age, height, and body build: small, medium, and large. They calculate with a range of eight to fifteen pounds what they think someone should weigh. Ten percent over that makes you overweight; 20 percent, and you are obese. This tolerance accords with the theory held by certain beauties that you look better, particularly in the face, if you let yourself flesh out a bit as you grow older. It works for some people but not for me. I would not get a smoother face; the added weight would go straight to the behind, and mine is big enough as it is. You have to know your physical type. "I'm really too small and skinny," says Louise (Loulou) de la Falaise, fashion consultant to Yves Saint Laurent, "but skinny people have a problem too, because they only put it on in the wrong place. If I thought eating was going to give me tits, I would eat the house down. Since it never does, it's pointless to force myself." The fact that most, though not all, women have a distribution problem explains the common acceptance on the beautiful people circuit of the five-pound limit rule.

The life insurance companies, of course, have a vested interest in longevity (don't you?). They contend that you should reach your desired weight at age twenty-five and stay there the rest of your life. I do not know why the magic age is twenty-five instead of twenty-one or twenty-eight. Ask them. I, for one, weighed more at age twenty-five than I do now because

I could carry it better then, and furthermore, it was only when I was into my thirties that the youth cult in fashion sent all my generation into a frantic contemplation of our thighs. Never underestimate the power of fashion for good as well as bad. The mini craze is dead, and the youth cult is on the wane, but pants and bikinis are here to stay, so this is no time to relax.

In practice the five-pound limit turns out to be less fanatic than it seems. There is a physiological reason why it is easier to lose weight as soon as it is gained.

Any medical student knows this. The explanation goes that when you first put on weight, the fat is still "soft" and high in water content. That is the time to lose it, before the body gets a chance to assimilate it. If you keep ten to fifteen pounds overweight on you for a year, it becomes part of the muscle structure. In other words, it marbelizes, as in fat steak, and is much harder to lose.

I do not gain any weight when following a normal routine, but what is normal? I have finally realized that business trips or a sudden jam-up of parties and eating out—perhaps at holiday time—are also part of the norm on a yearly basis and have to be reckoned with. At the magic number five a small inner voice scolds, "You're not really hungry. Don't eat so much. Just because the food's there is no reason to gorge." I listen, and usually within a few days I have lost the few pounds, the small voice is silent, and I want to eat again.

Often in such cases my technique is to eat my regular break-fast, about half my average lunch, skip dinner, and go to bed early with an apple and a book. To go to bed in a quiet room and feel snug helps take your mind off food. If you do not want to read, watch TV, though I must say that one of the unsung merits of reading is that it keeps your hands so busy that it's awkward to be messing about with food at the same time, especially in bed—you wind up with splotches on the book and crumbs in the sheets.

For keeping your weight stable, another quick method, if

your schedule permits, is a weekend or one-day fast. Rest for a day and eat nothing but apples or yogurt, or, if you can, drink only fruit juice, tea with honey, or just plain water. Mild activity is fine (when you get bored staying in bed), but mostly you should superorganize in advance so that your own or your family's practical needs have been catered to and you can retreat into a long dietetic laze—for twenty-four hours the world will have to spin by itself!

"If you can stay on vegetable boullion one day a week, it's marvelous for you," says Françoise de la Renta, wife of Oscar, the New York fashion designer. "You drink three quarts in twenty-four hours, preferably while resting, because lying down makes it more diuretic."

"When I have a weight problem," Merle Oberon says, "rather than cut down on everything, I simply live on yogurt, raisins, and almonds for a day or two. I add vitamins and protein powder to the yogurt."

"I don't diet, but buying larger clothes is such a bore that when I'm a few pounds over, I prefer to eat less," says Fiona Campbell Thyssen, former cover girl. "When one day of only fruit, one day of only meat, and one of salads doesn't do the trick, I get by on yogurt and honey. Or if I'm desperate, I just stop eating and lose those extra pounds that are making all my clothes hang wrong."

Out of curiosity, I have tried both mild and severe fasting and find both unpleasant. I do not mind skipping dinner, even enjoy it occasionally, but I like the rest of the day to proceed as usual (with smaller quantities, if necessary). Sitting down to nothing but clear soup or health food depresses me; it makes me feel like an invalid. There is one exception: when you are too tired or nervous to digest properly, a day in bed on liquids, fruit, or yogurt purifies the system. That it's slimming is an added bonus. This should not imply that a busy, active life makes you fat—it does not unless you keep busy eating—only that there are times when nervous fatigue is such that food intoxicates more than nourishes, and you need rest more than food (or another drink) to keep going.

An active life, with a supportable amount of stress, is, on the contrary, one of the keys to staying in shape. By active, I mean a combination of both mental and physical work and play. Marion Javits, wife of the New York senator, agrees: "Your sex life affects your maintenance." Or as Elaine Kennedy Gombault, London hostess and PR woman, states more flamboyantly: "I love to feel thin, and there's nothing like a new lover for that. The same old one won't do—after a while, you never lose a pound."

For keeping your weight in the right place, however, the standard answer is gymnastics and sports, touch football rather than "Touch." (Loulou de la Falaise explains that the latter starts when one partner says, "Let's go for a walk." The partners then proceed from "Go" to a fast hike around the bed. There are no other rules.) Unfortunately, for staying in shape nothing beats sportive sweat and spirit, unless it is the discipline of yoga or dance.

"You have to keep the joints loose and well lubricated," says Tamara Geva, former dancer and musical comedy star who left Russia with Balanchine when she was fifteen. "You have to make sure nothing grows in the back so you don't look humped over, and you watch out for the inner thighs. I've developed my own exercise routine which I follow regularly, because I know what makes each muscle work, but some movements are basic. If you begin to have a little pot belly, you suck it in and keep it in; when you walk, you pretend you have a gold coin between your buttocks; as for your hands, just play the piano.

"I have to give credit to God because I was born limber and the proportion was right (the only thing I didn't have was the neck). I really haven't changed since I was twenty—nothing hangs—and when I was about twenty in Hollywood, I had a figure to kill. No, I won't tell you how old I am, only that how you age depends to a certain extent on how you're built. If you're built right, it's easier to keep it."

"Staying busy keeps the body alive; my weight has been the same for fourteen years," says Janie Stevens, fashion magazine editor and wife of London *Daily Express* managing director Jocelyn Stevens. "I'm always working; I love chocolates and sweets, but I also love tennis and other sports. I never sit still. I have a real breakfast with bacon and eggs, orange juice, honey, and toast, but I never have huge meals, and I drink only wine. Four small meals a day are better for me than three large ones; I also try to eat very slowly."

"Moving keeps me thin," says London-based Georgiana Russell, journalist and daughter of the British ambassador to Spain. "I walk home from work, which I have clocked at twenty-nine minutes, including the lights. Once home, I often put records on and practice dance steps. The neighbors think I'm slightly loopy. As much as possible, I go to a dance studio here where one does a half hour's exercises to jazz; the teacher then improvises and one tries to follow the steps without knocking too many people down. It's a hangout for all sorts of types—a fabulous, scruffy, huge, and well-lit studio. And there's Tramp on a Friday night: jeans and easy shoes. You dance solidly for three hours and you lose four or five pounds. . . ."

Some of the above are English examples, but nationality has very little to do with it; what counts is attitude. When TV personality and London model school owner Cherry Marshall says briskly, "If your weight, give or take a few pounds, is right, you don't diet, you shape up with exercise," the comment applies to men and women anywhere, not just on a rainy island. I, for example, do not go dancing, nor do I swim much or play tennis. At home in Rome, I do what many of my New York friends rely on in Manhattan: I go to gym classes once a week. I also do what many Parisians do: I walk a lot.

"I go to the Bois every day with the two youngest children and the dogs," says Baroness Gaby van Zuylen. "We have a good hour's walk and we go early, though last year, when the Bois was full of joggers who drove off the satyrs, you could go whenever you wanted. Now that jogging has fallen off, the exhibitionists are back, and you have to avoid their prime time."

If you can exercise in big cities where you have to plan it, you can certainly exercise when you live in the country or suburbs, where you often have sports equipment in your own backyard.

"I used to swim in California, where it was easy because I had my own pool," says sculptor Marcia Panama. "When I first came to London, I tried exercise classes, but it cost a fortune and the classes got too crowded. I had qualms about visiting even the Grosvenor House pool because I am a pool snob. Theirs is sixty-five feet long and I must admit it's very pleasant. Ted Heath used to go to Grosvenor, Lady Morley and a few determined, strapping ladies go, plus lots of men in the film biz—you can't even get on the waiting list now.

"I'm there and back in forty-five minutes, unless it's a bad day for traffic. I go five days a week, and the point is, I really swim. I do my twenty lengths in twelve minutes. Exercise makes you feel marvelous and you become body-conscious on a subliminal level—you begin to stand straighter. During a trip to the States I went to have my legs waxed. The girl told me she knew I was a frequent swimmer; she could tell by the tone of my legs, and I wasn't even swimming regularly then. The other important thing about my swimming routine is that I haven't had to change my eating habits or diet."

The point is to care about energy, shape, and weight. Then, no matter where you are, find the time and the means to exercise. No one has to take you by the hand; feel the need and do it, even if it is just five minutes of stretching like a cat in bed every morning, as Arlene Dahl does "to tune up the motor."

You have to be aware, though, that exercise alone will not keep your weight down. It helps distribute it correctly and improves your measurements—with exercise the skirt that was getting tight around the waist feels comfortable again, maybe even loose. But to bring your weight in line and keep it there, the golden rule is to watch how and how much you eat. So long, starchy snacks; good-bye, sweet tooth; and down with haute cuisine!

I know the last sounds like heresy, and maybe it is! Haute cuisine is one of life's last luxuries and is marvelous to indulge in from time to time—when you pick up the staggering check, you are not just paying for a meal, you are paying a debt to civilization. On the other hand, who wants it every day? I cannot think of anyone whose weight has been right for years who enjoys a lot of complicated food and sauces. Most people find them killing. This is not to say that the guiding principles of good cooking—first-class basic ingredients, fresh produce, fine meat and fish—should be forsaken; it is the added touches and too many courses that do you in.

"I like French cooking," says Nicole Alphand, Pierre Cardin adviser and wife of the former French ambassador to the United States, "but I don't like complicated cooking. I adore pâté and a very good roast chicken, a first-rate fish with sauce mousseline, roast veal, pot au feu, ham with port sauce, and spinach. I always try to have fresh produce for the house. There's a cheese place on the rue de Grenelle where everyone goes, the rue Marbeuf for chicken, Avenue de la Grande Armée for beef—and Fauchon. You see I'm very *gourmande,* which means I should be given all the more credit for not getting fat."

"I like very light things," says American socialite Cappy
Badrutt of the Paris, St. Moritz, and international jet circuit.
"I don't like rich food, sauces, and sweets. I simply can't
handle them. I was at one of the Rothschilds' the other night
where the food was incredibly rich and the wines were the
best and the heaviest. You suffer! Fifty years ago you started
with caviar, terrapin soup, moved on to fish, fowl, and meat
with sorbet in between, and wound up with a savory. I wonder
how people survived. Now you can still eat well, but you
simplify, and when you travel you look for the little local foods
rather than elaborate dishes."

For my part, while I refuse to be browbeaten by the myth
of haute cuisine, I certainly do not think, as has been claimed,
that American food is the best and most nutritious in the
world. In fact, I am appalled to see the copycat industrializa-
tion of food in Europe. For my pleasure as well as my figure,
I try to defend what is left of the middle ground between the
lofty, overbearing plateau of haute cuisine and the abyss of
overprocessed convenience foods. Joan Kennedy startled me
when she said that, left to her own devices, without her French
chef, she found cooking for herself on her own so boring that
she's capable of opening a can of chicken à la king and a can
of spaghetti and eating them cold. Prefab spaghetti makes my
blood run cold, and I would never have a can of chicken à la
king in the house! At the same time, I would never order coq
au vin or duck à l'orange. My idea of bird is broiled or roasted
with a few herbs. That is what I mean by the middle ground:
good, simple food.

"I think most people in the United States don't know what
they're eating," says Ceezee Guest. "I have been aware of
what is fattening all my life, and I never eat it—I can't stand
fried food, and I always have sauces served separately. When
the children eat with me, we never put tons of butter on food.
I like meat: I was brought up to eat roast beef, steak, and lamb
chops. Meat is what gives you strength and energy. I have

vegetables from the garden, and I love fruit. I adore it. I am not a dessert person. I never take sugar in coffee. For energy I often eat protein toast with honey and I have honey with my tea."

You eat superbly at Ceezee's house. You eat superbly at Cristina Ford's. American food can be among the best and most nutritious in the world if you know how to prepare it and exclude all the instant junk—when I go into a supermarket, my first reaction is: "That's not food, that's packaging." The quantity and variety are incredible and, to my mind, totally unnecessary.

"The food I like is basic," says Cristina Ford. "Even if I'm having a dinner party, I won't serve anything complicated— no French sauces, nothing 'special,' unless you call special having everything perfectly fresh.

"When I travel, I, like everyone, tend to overeat, especially in Italy. At home I start the day with fresh fruit. I adore having grapes or peaches in the morning instead of juice. How can you mix orange juice with tea? It gives you such an acid stomach! Then I have two pieces of wheat bread with one fresh boiled egg and my gossip tea with honey. That's about eleven o'clock, so I skip lunch, or maybe I have some fruit and cheese around two o'clock. Then I have a big dinner at night, fresh fish and a lot of vegetables. That is not very much."

In her own quite personal way, Cristina exemplifies how to eat well and stay thin. She thinks it is in her nature to go to bone rather than fat as she grows older but is not about to trust nature alone. Splurges are in her character—on the one hand, the food orgy with friends at a favorite restaurant, or the vanishing act with a box of chocolates; on the other, the total fast in bed, with only a drop of water, which became, until she lost her will, a one-day-a-week habit. Between these two extremes lies her regular Grosse Pointe regimen of fresh, simple food, two meals and one snack a day, along with two hours of gym and ballet (the house is equipped for both), biking around the neighborhood, and five-mile walks. Rest assured, her weight gain never exceeds the five-pound limit!

I do not suggest you doggedly copy her regimen, or anyone else's. Satisfactory long-term eating and exercise habits have to be individual or you will not stick to them. Ceezee Guest eats more than I do; Janet Leigh, when it is hot, lunches on a shake of ice cream and Metrecal, which would never occur to me. I feel fine with nothing but tea and honey for breakfast, which may be one reason I need a real lunch. I know that, in theory, a good breakfast with protein is important, but I think it is even more important to eat only when you feel like it. If I suddenly started to get the midmorning queasies, I would switch to more at breakfast and less at midday. I am a mineral water fiend like most beautiful people; in my case, it's because I drink very few other liquids. Alcohol is poison to my liver, although I do have wine or champagne when I go out. Marion Javits tells me that her husband, on the contrary, cannot touch red wine because that is his poison. "Each chemistry is different," she adds; she limits her fruit and vegetable intake to artichokes, asparagus, tomatoes, avocados, and grapefruit to combat water retention. For me, cutting out salt does the trick.

It really comes down to using your head as well as following your personal inclinations. Once you have eliminated the garbage, both lowbrow and haute—packaged gimcrack and superrich stuffing and sauces—and opted for simpler food, what you eat most of, animal or vegetable, and how you distribute your feeding during the day are really up to you. Your energy level, scales, and mirror soon tell you if you are right. I know what works for me. I have listed it below in the form of menus for any average week when I am home and can choose exactly what I want. Quite obviously, this is not what I eat every week; it is just an example. I do not weigh the portions, nor do I count the calories. What I eat is what the family eats, in larger or smaller portions, and the family, barring school and business absences, now consists of Mama Bear, Papa Bear, and five (God help us!) teen-agers.

Monday

Breakfast: 7:30–8:00 A.M.	1/2 grapefruit (Substitute an orange, fresh pineapple, peaches, or any other fruit you love to bite into first thing in the morning. Mostly I find delight in counting on my grapefruit.) Tea with slice of lemon (which I eat) and honey
Lunch: 1:30 P.M.	Shredded carrot vinaigrette Assorted cheeses or a piece of broiled lean meat Fruit
Dinner: 8:00 P.M.	Spaghetti with tomato sauce and basil (or cheese and butter) Salad vinaigrette (see comments at end of menus) Fruit

Tuesday

Breakfast	Same
Lunch	Crêpes au gratin Salad Fruit
Dinner	Chicken breasts (usually breaded and fried or sautéed and sprinkled with parsley) Salad Fruit

Wednesday

Breakfast   Same

Lunch   Veal scallopini with lemon
Roast potato
Salad
Fruit

Dinner   Pizza
Salad
Fruit

Thursday

Breakfast   Same

Lunch   Steak or roast beef
Salad

Dinner   Assorted cheeses
Ham or other cold cuts
Fruit

Friday

Breakfast   Same

Lunch   Tripe with rice
Salad

Dinner   Assorted cheeses
Fruit

Saturday

Breakfast   Same

Lunch   Liver marinated in soy sauce with lemon
Boiled potatoes

Salad

Fruit

Dinner   Spaghetti alla carbonara or with four-cheese
                 sauce
             Salad
             Fruit

Sunday

Breakfast   Same

Lunch   Hamburger
              Mashed potatoes
              Salad

Dinner   Eggplant Parmesan
              Salad
              Fruit

The menu has an Italian flavor—I live in Rome and further-more I think you are happier respecting your origins in food. (In my late teens, when I hated the way I looked, I went on a meat-salad-fruit binge so severe that I was doubled over with stomach pains. I stubbornly ignored them as long as I could—how could I have an ulcer from eating such healthy foods? Subsequent consultations with the family doctor re-vealed no lesion, only a need for a minimum daily supplement of olive oil and pasta, bread, or rice, which I thought was a terribly old-fashioned, ignorant diagnosis. As it turned out, the doctor was right. It was ignorant of me to forget the conditioning of an Italian background, and what he was tell-ing me was to add some fat and carbohydrates to a basically protein, vitamin, and mineral diet. In North America or northern Europe the doctor might have talked in terms of potatoes, bread, and butter.) The menu includes more car-bohydrates than yours might because high-protein fare does not agree with me. I never have meat more than once a day except when there are leftovers I am too frugal to waste (I'd rather spend saved pennies on other fillips). However, I do get additional protein from cheese. I do not snack, though in between meals I drink water or may have tea or fruit juice in the late afternoon. Wine is there for the asking at meals; I sometimes have some with dinner.

When my husband is home, I may have a bit of his pastry as a breakfast supplement or find a few spoonfuls of the yogurt/wheat germ/muesli/blackstrap molasses mix he believes in thrust down my throat. I eat cheese without bread but do sometimes use country (never white) bread as a pusher with meals. No frozen foods, no canned goods, with the possible exception of peeled tomatoes, sardines, and tuna. Fruit depends on the seasons. When tired of the more restricted winter selection, I supplement with dried fruits and nuts.

Fresh green salad never palls as far as I am concerned, and I see no reason for special dressings when olive oil, salt, pepper, lemon juice, and wine vinegar exist. Obviously, you vary the salad greens according to season and/or other availability: lettuce, romaine, chicory, watercress, endive, *rugula,* field salad. In some cases, add a few leaves of basil, *rughetta,* or tarragon, substitute wine vinegar for lemon, use a different oil if you must—I do prefer olive oil with salad. Throw in chopped celery, fennel, sliced cucumber, or tomato if you have them at hand and feel the urge. Slice in a leftover boiled potato or a hard-cooked egg. Apart from this basic routine, everyone has her special salads. A few of mine are:

Carrot, raw spinach, and *rugula* with bacon
Corn, avocado, Swiss cheese, and lettuce
Tomato, mozzarella cheese, and basil
Raw artichokes (dip in olive oil, salt, and pepper)
Carrot, avocado, tomato, Swiss cheese, and endive

I find this sort of eating pattern both filling and enjoyable, and the family has yet to complain. You may think, "My God, I'd be starving if I tried that." I can assure you that, at five feet seven and 127 pounds, I am not undernourished.

Just a reminder: Eve Arnold, the photographer, once did a spread on how the beautiful women of France kept fit. She took pictures of mistresses and duchesses on bicycles, doing yoga, or "le footing," which was all well and good but still did not really explain their slenderness. Finally, one of them turned to her and said, "I'll tell you what it is. We don't eat very much."

A Note on Cellulite— ### the Orange Peel Syndrome

The ugliest fat is not always necessarily overweight. You can be perfectly proportioned, even have a model's figure, and still be afflicted with cellulite. It looks like orange rind when squeezed and usually develops first on the back of the upper thighs. It spreads both downward and to the sides, and in the end you wind up with a rear sprawl that is known in the beauty trade as riding breeches.

Cellulite can also form on other areas of the thighs, the knees, ankles, upper arms, and the back of the neck. It is by no means fatal and, unless accompanied by obesity, constitutes no recognized menace to health. Nonetheless, like all women bothered by it, I am convinced that anything that looks that bad cannot be good for you.

So far I continue to stave it off with brisk manual tactics, the theory behind this being that cellulite is the result of bad circulation. Not only do I rely on my gym instructor, who uses heat lamps followed by strong massage, I follow up at home with towel flagellations twice a week. Supposedly, one should alternate hot with cold, but I have found cold alone most effective and use a wrung-out towel fresh out of the freezer. A good swat makes the cellulite zone pink and glowing, and for three days the incipient lumpy surface becomes smooth. Then I swat again.

My measures are mostly preventive and might do more harm than good in an advanced, flabby case of cellulite. An alternate manual approach is the specialty of French clinics, such as those at Trouville and Quiberon. It consists of hot baths of seawater laced with algae reinforced with underwater massage and other hydrotherapy.

The French have also pioneered in medical research on cellulite, influencing doctors elsewhere to reevaluate the problem instead of dismissing it as a purely cosmetic concern. This new thinking was triggered by the fact that men rarely have cellulite whereas women almost always do—a slight amount of it can be classed as a secondary sex characteristic in women. While not a sickness in itself, cellulite is now regarded as a possible symptom of endocrine, metabolic, or functional disorder.

Doctors Pierre Dukan and Michel Pistor, for example, suspect that an excess of estrogen may be a cause and suggest restoring hormonal balance as the basis of a cure for cellulite when tests reveal an estrogen excess. However, not all women with orange-peel ankles and riding-breech bottoms are hyper-estrogen. Some other reason must be found to explain water retention and cellulite. Heredity, stress, diet, poor breathing habits, and functional disorders such as lordosis and flat feet have been named in the general search to find a culprit.

Pistor proposes localized multi-injections and Dukan suggests ionization to disperse cellulite formation. Both oppose strong massage as being harmful to veins and capillaries; furthermore, by "breaking down" the nodules and detaching them from the muscle, one risks transforming a firm cellulite into a floating glob. After medical treatment—multi-injections or ionization—mild massage is recommended to stimulate circulation.

Ionization is done by applying to the cellulite zones plates wrapped in sponge soaked in a mix of products such as enzymes, thyroid extract, and heparin. The plates are wired to a medium-frequency generator, which is then switched on. The electric current causes local penetration of the products. As for the multi-injection method, seven to eighteen needles inject a total of 40 cc of a similar cocktail—20 cc per upper thigh. It hurts, although the needles are much shorter than those used individually for any normal shot. The cocktail might include procaine at 2 percent, thyroid extract, heparin, and possibly iodine, artichoke extract, and gonadotrophin (so one Roman practitioner, Dr. Carlo Alberto Bartoletti, tells me).

I have never tried either method, although I do have friends who are enthusiastic about them. Even if a multi-injection with short needles affects only a superficial area, I confess I would have to have a lot of cellulite to undergo one—40 cc of anything is enough to stagger a horse.

At present multi-injections including procaine are not recognized in the United States. Until something else is invented, you will have to go along with whatever form of massage makes most sense to you. Meanwhile, if you have cellulite, there are certain practical things you can do. The first is to throw out your girdle, garter belt, or anything else you wear that cuts both your skin and circulation. The second regards diet. Check with your doctor, but try and keep salt and salty foods at a minimum, along with sweets, tobacco, and alcohol.

3

Take It Off

The shock usually comes at the turn of the season when you try on a bathing suit. You discover to your dismay that you are not the size and shape you used to be. So that is why your clothes have been feeling tight! Ten to twenty pounds have crept up on you, a burden that both your looks and your health could do without. You want to get rid of them, that is for sure, because what looks bad in the mirror is not going to look any better on the beach, even with a tan.

The first question you ask is: How fast can I lose? The answer is up to you: not overnight, which is everyone's dream, but certainly within a month to a year depending on the technique you use and on how much you have to shed. (Ten pounds move faster than twenty.) One would like to think that excess body fat could just melt away like the ice cream, chocolate, and butter that helped cause it, except that body fat does not work that way. Wishing will not make it go; diet will.

Nevertheless, it's not how fast you lose but how long the weight stays lost that counts. Supervised fasting or one of any number of stringent diets will cut you down to size and may be necessary as an initial tactic. If you then revert to the eating pattern that made you fat, the pounds roll right back on. Obesity specialist Dr. Neil Solomon calls this the Yo-Yo syndrome. It is also known as the seesaw, the Scotch shower, and the expanding theory of the universe.

The only advantage to crash dieting is that you see the weight slip off you—deprivation brings a tangible reward. But without reeducation, the reward turns out to be a booby prize, and you have to diet again. Nonetheless, I can see why people do it. It is useless to preach nutrition to someone whose prime concern is how to look great for an imminent party, wedding, or vacation. Many crash diets, while ineffectual in the overall campaign, are harmless as long as you follow them for only a few weeks. (No one in her right mind would prolong the agony.) Women's magazines and the women's page of any newspaper are loaded with these diets. As far as I am concerned, go ahead and try one, if you must, as long as you realize you are only resorting to a stop-gap device.

After you abandon the crash diet, there is always the chance that you will retain some sensible habit that limits weight. For example, after ten days of drinking coffee black or eating grapefruit without sugar, you may discover to your surprise that you like them better that way.

One word of warning: there is a circumstance in which you cannot play around, and that is when overweight is associated with a diagnosed illness. In the case of any malfunction that is aggravated by fat, your doctor will insist you take off weight, and he will regulate the speed. Having to reduce because of impaired health is not the same as reducing by choice, and obviously you must follow your doctor's instructions, however impalatable. At most, if you cannot stand the diet he prescribes, shop around for another doctor who may have one you prefer that is equally suitable for your condition. Nutrition is not an exact science with immutable formulas. On the other hand, if you have a health problem, your dieting should be supervised. You should try to keep informed on pertinent new thinking, but you cannot afford the risk of experimenting on your own with diets, however appealing, that may upset your system even more.

Assuming instead that your only problem is that you're growing unpleasingly plump, I pass on the diet below as an example of one way to lose weight fast and still go about your business. It is austere but balanced. At worst, it could make you a social recluse.

I also use it to illustrate a point. Most of us find diets passed on to us by some enthusiastic friend more compelling than something we read about, clip, and never try. (The printed page does not check on you as a friend does.) We fall for the diet even more when the person who talks about it obviously has lost weight and looks ravishing. Fashion designer Vera Maxwell, known for her superb clothes for the country club set, had the following formula pressed upon her by just such a crusading lady friend—the sort you may encounter tomorrow at a party, in the office, or around the sandbox, anyplace where women swap news. The point is that Mrs. Maxwell asked for a more qualified opinion before she leaped. I recommend this though sometimes I wonder why, in view of most doctors' astonishing ineptitude at curing overweight.

"I find diets dull because you have to give up your social life," Mrs. Maxwell says, "but I feel marvelous when I do this one, which a friend gave me. It's an elimination diet. My son is a doctor, and he told me, 'If you must go on a trick diet, Mother, this one's OK.'"

WEEKLY ELIMINATION DIET

Day 1

Breakfast   5 ounces orange or grapefruit juice
1 cup dry cereal with a little skimmed milk
(about 1/2 cup) and
honey (2 tsp.)
2 slices dry toast
1 cup mint tea (optional)

Lunch   2 eggs Florentine (1 medium portion spinach)
on 1 slice dry toast
3 pieces celery
4 tablespoons applesauce
5 ounces skimmed milk

Dinner   2 small broiled lamb chops (fat trimmed) or 1
medium hamburger
medium portion steamed asparagus or any
green vegetable
1 medium baked potato
5 stewed apricots or prunes

Bedtime   5 ounces orange or grapefruit juice or
skimmed milk

Day 2

Breakfast   5 ounces orange or grapefruit juice
2 slices dry toast
5 ounces skimmed milk
1 cup mint tea (optional)

Lunch   1 egg Florentine on 1 slice dry toast
4 tablespoons applesauce
5 ounces skimmed milk

Dinner   1 broiled lamb chop or 1 small hamburger

medium portion steamed asparagus or any
green vegetable

4 tablespoons strawberries or raspberries,
preferably stewed

Bedtime 5 ounces of orange or grapefruit juice or
skimmed milk

Day 3

Breakfast 5 ounces orange or grapefruit juice
1 slice dry toast
5 ounces skimmed milk
1 cup mint tea (optional)

Lunch 1 medium portion spinach
4 tablespoons applesauce

Dinner medium portion green vegetable
4 tablespoons fruit

Bedtime 5 ounces of orange or grapefruit juice or
skimmed milk

Day 4

Breakfast, lunch, dinner, bedtime: choice of 5 ounces
orange or grapefruit
juice or skimmed milk

Day 5

Repeat Day 3

Day 6

Repeat Day 2

Day 7

Repeat Day 1

Throughout, you have no coffee, tea (except for mint tea, which is optional), or liquor. This is important, because you disintoxicate yourself as well as reduce. You should drink 2 full glasses of water per day. Ideally, you begin the diet on Thursday so that Day 4, when you fast, falls on a restful Sunday. Mrs. Maxwell, who is a sensationally attractive grandmother, says that she feels marvelous when she goes on the diet and loses at least four pounds: "I don't know why I don't do it more often," she said. "I suppose it's because I have a business to run."

For more gradual loss, the next diet is a modification of the classic one-of-a-kind repetition formula: one day meat, one day fruit, and so on. This version, planned by Rome's Dr. Alberto Lodispoto, is not so extreme and is easy to follow whether you eat in or out. At the 1,200 to 1,400 calorie level, you should lose about two pounds every ten days. The higher calorie levels are for maintenance. Below is the basic form of the diet; sample menus follow.

Breakfast	Only fruit
10–11 A.M.	A little fruit if hungry
Lunch	*Food you can eat:* bread, pasta, rice, potatoes, beans, lentils light tomato sauce a bit of fat (butter, oil, margarine for the sauce) raw or cooked vegetables 1 glass of dry wine *Foods to avoid:* eggs, cheese, milk, cream *Forbidden food:* meat, fish, fats, sauces, fruit
4–5 P.M.	A little fruit if hungry

Dinner   *Foods you can eat:*
              meat, fish, eggs, cheese, fresh salad in abun-
                 dance
              1 glass dry wine
              Foods to avoid:
              flour, bread, rice, white sauce
              Forbidden food:
              bread, breadsticks, crackers, pasta, rice,
                 potatoes, beans, lentils, and fruit

Throughout the diet, do not take tea, coffee, cocoa, chocolate drinks, sugar, honey, jam or jelly, syrups, or any pastry
or sweets.

Approximately 1,200 Calories

Breakfast   1 glass fresh orange juice (5 ounces)

Midmorning   an apple or a pear

Lunch   pasta or rice (3 ounces, uncooked)
              tomatoes (3 ounces)
              oil (2 tablespoons)
              raw vegetables (3 1/2 ounces), with dress-
                 ing of a little of the oil, salt, and lemon
                 juice
              potatoes (4 ounces)
              1 glass dry wine (4 ounces)

Midafternoon an apple or a pear

Dinner   1 cup (8 ounces) consommé (with the fat
                 skimmed off)
              broiled lean veal (3 1/2 ounces), or fish (5
                 ounces), poached, broiled, or steamed
              1 egg, or low-fat cheese (2 ounces)
              salad or raw vegetables (3 1/2 ounces),
                 with a little oil, salt, and lemon juice
              1 glass dry wine (4 ounces)

Approximately 1,400 Calories

Breakfast	1 glass fresh orange juice (5 ounces)
Midmorning	an apple or a pear
Lunch	pasta or rice (3 1/2 ounces) tomatoes (3 1/2 ounces) oil (2 tablespoons) salad or raw vegetables (3 1/2 ounces), with a little of the oil, salt, and lemon juice potatoes (5 ounces) 1 glass dry wine (4 ounces)
Midafternoon	an apple or a pear
Dinner	1 cup (8 ounces) consommé (with the fat skimmed off) lean veal (3 1/2 ounces), or fish (5 ounces) 1 egg, or low-fat cheese (2 ounces) salad or raw vegetables (3 1/2 ounces), with a little oil, salt, and lemon juice 1 glass dry wine (4 ounces)

Approximately 1,600 Calories

Breakfast	1 glass fresh orange juice (5 ounces)
Midmorning	an apple or a pear
Lunch	pasta or rice (4 ounces) tomatoes (3 1/2 ounces) oil (2 1/2 tablespoons) potatoes (5 ounces) bread (2 ounces) raw vegetables or salad (3 1/2 ounces), with a little of the oil, salt, and lemon juice 1 glass dry wine (4 ounces)

Midafternoon an apple or a pear

Dinner 1 cup (8 ounces) consommé (with the fat skimmed off)
lean veal (5 ounces), or fish (7 ounces)
1 egg, or low-fat cheese (2 ounces)
salad or raw vegetables (3 1/2 ounces), with a little oil, salt, and lemon juice
1 glass dry wine (4 ounces)

Approximately 1,800 Calories

Breakfast 1 glass fresh orange juice (5 ounces)

Midmorning an apple or a pear

Lunch pasta or rice (5 ounces)
tomatoes (5 ounces)
oil (2 1/2 tablespoons)
potatoes (5 ounces)
bread (2 ounces)
salad or raw vegetables (3 1/2 ounces), with a little of the oil, salt, and lemon juice
1 glass dry wine (4 ounces)

Midafternoon an apple or a pear

Dinner 1 cup (8 ounces) consommé (with fat skimmed off)
lean veal (5 ounces), or fish (7 ounces)
1 egg, or low-fat cheese (3 ounces)
salad or raw vegetables (3 1/2 ounces), with oil (2 tablespoons), a little salt, and lemon juice
1 glass dry wine (4 ounces)

On the whole, though I have listed two of them, I question whether any standardized diet is the solution to overweight, unless by chance you hit upon one that seems made to order for you. We are dealing here with a flux of ten to twenty pounds, which is by no means ingrained obesity. Such a shift reflects bad eating habits and may even indicate a mild neurosis, but it does not imply any fierce emotional hangup about food. At the same time, ten to twenty pounds can be most depressing, particularly when they keep coming back despite your repeated efforts.

"I'm a happier person when I'm thinner," says bright, pretty Jori Pepper, now working in educational TV and the daughter of writer Curtis G. (Bill) Pepper and sculptor Beverly. "I'm surer of myself. When you wake up heavy, all you want to do is roll over and go back to sleep."

In the course of five years, Jori, who is now twenty-one, tried a half-dozen diets, two of them with specialists and the others on her own. Does that sound familiar? It is the old Yo-Yo syndrome again, and if you have ever spun up and down in weight, you know exactly how she feels. Her vicissitudes illustrate the diet quandary remarkably well and point to one way out.

Encouraged to lose a little weight when she was sixteen, Jori felt deprived and began to get fat, took the Simeons cure (see chapter 4), lost twenty-two pounds in a month and stayed at a stable weight until, as she expresses it, she got unhappy. Still, her next real bout with overweight didn't start until a few years later when she left Rome, where she grew up, and Paris, where she studied, for New York. Jori is American, but she was not prepared for the national food marathon.

"Suddenly I had to choose from so many different kinds of non-foods—all those fattening snacks," she says. "The meal hours are too crammed together, and when you eat out, you get such huge portions. The culture is geared to food, with ads for cakes and cookies splashed on every wall. You can eat all night in a city like New York, and they'll even deliver dinners right to your door. The deli in our building is open seven days a week, twenty-four hours a day, and the city is made up of all the big eaters: the Jews love to eat, as do the Italians and the Germans. . . . But it isn't just the ethnic eating; the ice cream market in New York is enormous. Baskin-Robbins will put you on their mailing list and send you the announcement of each month's flavors. You cannot imagine the sensuality of going in there. The ice cream is truly spectacular, and they let you taste everything. Gael Greene did a cover story for *New York* magazine on ice cream in which she described how she waited and waited her turn while a little boy tried every flavor. He finally took vanilla, and her comment was: 'There was a kid with real problems.'

"The irony is that the whole ideal in America is to be rich and slim. I wonder whether a lot of people aren't fat because there's so much pressure to be thin. Supermarkets have whole departments of diet food and drink—it's almost easier to find low-cal products than regular, while the point is that no one needs to eat and drink all that much. It's just insane. I mean, there's something wrong about a nation where it's considered foolish to eat real butter because you're wasting calories."

Among the diets Jori tried on her own were a brown rice diet and total fasting. The rice trip (of macrobiotic persuasion) gave her splitting headaches, and when she started eating regular foods again, she found that her attitude toward food had not changed at all. In other words, she still ate more than she could burn up. In Bridgehampton, where she was cooking for a household of ten people, she went on a ten-day fast, which, may I add, I do not recommend that anyone do on his own. Fasting prevented her from tasting to correct seasoning, but she got so she could smell when the food was too salty—"it's amazing and very exciting how the senses develop.

"The smell of New York when I first went back was like

dead fish stuffed up my nose. The first thing I ate," she says, "was tuna fish, and the metallic taste was overwhelming. I tried to drink a glass of soda. It was disgusting."

Unfortunately, she had not lost either very much weight or her fattening habits when she went back to eating. Diuretics? Yes, she flirted with those too, noting that they make you feel twenty pounds lighter until the moment you have a drink of water and puff up. Her moment of truth came when she went to one of the leading New York reducing doctors.

"His diets are supposed to be tailored to your needs," she says. "To start with, you drink glucose and have about twelve blood tests in four hours that cost you $120, so you figure you're going to get something different from the diet of his that was published in a magazine. I wanted to lose twenty pounds, the average there is forty. His associate explained that they would find my danger foods, but he talked about personal treatment in such an impersonal way, it could have been a record.

"After ten days, I went back to get the results and paid another $20 or $30 to have my chart analyzed in great detail, except that the associate admitted he'd never seen a glucose reaction like mine and didn't know how to deal with it. He then gave me a mimeographed slip of paper with a diet identical to the published one—it was filled in differently on coffee. You're supposed to use only his sweetener. I found another one like his on the market—one that metabolizes like protein rather than carbohydrate—and it cost less. His only reason why I shouldn't use it? 'Because I said no.'

"You're supposed to report back every week to weigh in, and you find all those wealthy women there—the kind who need to be slapped on the wrist and lectured because they've cheated. The doctor's bill forms are so big, they look like a bank statement—there's enough room for a year of visits. I got so mad that I pulled myself together and finally started eating sensibly on my own."

There are several aspects of this diet morality tale that

cannot be stressed enough, which is why I have quoted it at length. The first one is that intelligent curiosity and a willingness to experiment are as important in attacking overweight as they are in dealing with any other problem. Finding your limit with food is one facet of finding yourself. Sometimes, as happened with Jori, outrage can be the best prompter, and "I'll show them," the strongest motivation.

Secondly, please note that thousands of women have tried the same New York doctor and many continue with his method and are pleased with the results. With diets, what works for one person turns the next one off, and rightly so, because our physical, emotional, and aesthetic needs are not the same. If you are lucky and hit the right doctor and the right diet, you may never have to go through the process of thinking out your own personal regimen.

When Jori met her husband, he was about thirty-five pounds overweight, and it was his first trip to Paris. In the circumstances, she found it really very sweet of him to comply when she said he had to lose weight. He went on a fashionable high-protein diet, slimmed within a few weeks, and has not gained a pound since.

"He's twenty-five, five feet eleven or something, and he's thin. He eats huge quantities of food, but it's all protein," she says. "He hardly ever eats fruit or vegetables. When he eats fruit, he feels guilty. He eats meat, fish, hard and soft cheese, and eggs. I'm getting him to eat lettuce now. We never drink booze, though I must say it's such fun when I go back to Rome, to drink wine."

Good for him if he likes it and feels well. You, on the other hand, may have a strong vegetarian streak or really feel the need for your daily bread. If you prefer to use some standard impersonal diet, it is only common sense for you to choose one close to your inclinations. Unless you do, the effects of your shock-troop attack on overweight will never carry over into a stabilized routine.

Glamorous Joanne King, Houston TV personality, sums

this idea up perfectly. Diet is one of the more popular topics on her show.

"You can eat a mountain of celery and cottage cheese, but sometimes it is better to eat half of what you prefer, even when it is cake or other forbidden goodies. Too much boring diet food often results in an eating binge. Feeling psychologically satisfied after eating is important. This is the cause, I feel, of most dieters' failure. They become so weary of never enjoying what they are told they should eat that they lose their incentive."

I could not agree more. Better to add protein powder or vitamin-mineral supplements, as the need may be, to any reasonable eating pattern that keeps you satisfied and thin, than to force yourself to obey diet dictates that strike you as both arbitrary and repellent.

Which brings me to point three of our diet morality tale: the flavorless land of plenty. While I approve of nutrition supplements, the pseudo-convenience of snacking and stuffing on super-processed packaged foods strikes me as absurd. How can you limit intake on the instinctive basis of taste preference, when everything tastes the same?

When you live in America, perhaps you become inured. Coming to the States from abroad for a visit, however, you are overwhelmed by billboard, neon, television, and magazine ads for factory food. The sandwich is so popular in America that you feel you are wrapped in bread twenty-four hours a day. If you venture into a supermarket, you are totally stunned by the plethora of goods that are identifiable only by pasted-on picture or label—no touch, no smell, no see, except, at best, dimly through a tiny plastic window. Add to prefab basics the hundreds of prepared sauces, condiments, and salad dressings, and no wonder you get fat; you cannot even tell what you are eating.

Personally, I do not know anyone among my American friends who buys this stuff. I assume, though, because of its abundance, that there must be a huge market and that cooking has been replaced by exercises in mechanics: carving metal, pulling strings and tabs, squeezing cardboard, tearing on dotted lines, and punching holes. On the other hand, where weight, taste, nutrition, and even time are concerned, the real convenience foods are milk, cheese, eggs, fruit, salad, whole-grain bread, lean meat, innards, and fish. Nor are they necessarily more expensive.

"If the American public would go back to the diet as it was thirty years ago, there is no question but that we would use, with the same income that we have, a substantially smaller proportion of the family budget. . . . However, if the majority of American housewives would go back to the more simple diet of thirty years ago, the result would be an appalling collapse in the food industry," Dr. Karl Brandt, A.G.R., pointed out in the 1966 Voice of America Symposium on Food and Civilization.

One of the most dubious recent innovations is the flood of special diet foods. A few do make sense, such as using a salt substitute when regular salt is taboo for health reasons. The same goes for artificial sweeteners. But why on earth buy a package of diet food when fresh food is no more fattening, often costs less, and tastes better? According to Peter Wyden, author of *The Overweight Society*, "Even when people have used low-calorie products for some time, there is no evidence that this has helped many of them to a trimmer figure."

"Economically speaking, diet foods are a disaster . . . except for a handful of products . . ." writes Jennifer Cross in *The Supermarket Trap*. "The food industry is well aware that we all have our little weaknesses, and sees to it that they cost us money. The weight watcher—about one person in four—is high up on this sucker list. She increasingly looks to diet foods, many of which are more expensive than their full-calorie equivalent, as a substitute for strength of mind, and is often misled by phoney claims of misleading labels."

Strength of mind? Willpower? However you choose to define it, if you are overweight, it too is flabby, and a serious reckoning is in order. I, for one, think that a compulsion to check the fat at ten to twenty pounds is already a positive sign. Why not go one step further and give up gimmick foods and crash diets once and for all, especially as the results have never lasted for long?

As a final point, I suggest that you sit yourself down, favorite snack at hand for moral support, and reevaluate your eating pattern. Adhering to any one of the hundreds of diets available depends, in the last analysis, on your will to do so. Since that's the case, you might as well figure out your own scheme. The idea is not new but have you ever done it? To provide raw material, you start by listing day by day everything you eat and drink for a week—no one is going to scold you, so you might as well be honest. "Everything" includes, for instance, how many spoonfuls of sugar. On your list, with the days of the week on the left, place your food and drink in columns under five basic headings: dairy products, meat and other proteins, vegetables and fruits, fats, and carbohydrate products. Some duplication is inevitable: cheese is both dairy and protein; butter both dairy and fat; potatoes carbohydrate, but the butter or oil you use with them is fat. When it comes to processed foods, you are in trouble; I would suggest adding an extra column entitled "garbage."

Quite obviously, the purpose of this chart is to give you an overall view of your habits. If you have a weight problem, the odds are that carbohydrates and garbage will dominate with fats running a close third. Rather than swear off all of them, the trick is selectivity. Which starches, fats, and sweet things are indispensable to your joy in life and which can you do without? A lot! Chic, weight-conscious Françoise de la Renta, for example, reserves the right to one chocolate a day. Someone else might forgo candy to allow himself a drink. Take away pasta, and I would die, which means that I barely touch bread. He who loves bacon cuts down on other animal fats. All I am saying is that something has to give, and it need not be your waistline.

If you want, consult a calorie booklet to refresh your memory on the most and least fattening items in the various food categories. Calories do count, and the only reason I do not suggest you tally them is that with just overweight, rather than obesity, the essential to grasp is that starches, sweets, fried foods, sauces, salty extras, soft drinks, and liquor are the enemy. They will be the victorious enemy unless you divide, knock off most of them, and conquer.

Monitoring yourself does not always bring quick results. It takes a while to learn just how much to cut back, but hopefully the pounds that you gradually lose will stay lost. Depending on the degree of your addiction to sweets, be prepared to miss eating and drinking them as you start cutting back, maybe even for months, although withdrawal symptoms should not be too drastic if you allow yourself a special favorite. After a while, you will really wonder what you saw in them.

Again, as Joanne King told me: "In my experience, the absence of sweets or breads in my daily diet makes a great difference simply because without these two I am not tempted to have just a little snack. The snack I could have (raw vegetables, for example) is not as readily available as a cracker or a cookie, nor do raw vegetables taste as good."

One important note: As you start eating less, stay as active as before, more so if possible, because if you sit around, the body will adjust and you will hardly lose a pound.

It is all up to you—who else? Obviously, if you had a disease, I would say to go to a doctor and pay for his skill, but when you are healthy, and it's just a matter of ten to twenty pounds, I confess I would rather be stingy. I would not pay thirty to fifty dollars a consultation, much less undergo shock therapy or hypnotism for what I could do myself. Once you have drawn up your chart and begin to see what your worse habits are, the following general suggestions will help you structure a new eating pattern, one that satisfies you and keeps you slim.

1) I am geared to a light breakfast and two meals plus tea or fresh fruit juice at midafternoon. In between, food is out of sight, out of mind. I never snack. If you, on the contrary, function better by eating more often, do it, just as long as you eat less at regular mealtimes. The point is to find your own pace. For example, if you cannot bear the thought of eating breakfast but also cannot make it through to lunch without feeling weak, get yourself organized. Have your coffee or tea, which is all you want when you first get up, then an hour or so later take a break for a piece of bread, meat, cheese, or a hard-cooked egg and fruit. (Bring it to the office, if necessary.) At lunchtime have a light lunch, which is all you will need. I say this because if the pit of your stomach goes queasy mid-morning, you are going to reach for something, and it might as well be low-cal and nutritious instead of some ghastly sweet bun washed down with sugary coffee and cream.

2) Are you always thirsty? How about reaching for water, with or without a squeeze of lemon? I am not a water fetishist; I do not think my kidneys will collapse if I don't drink four glasses a day, but when I am thirsty, water is the "soft drink" for me. During meals, to avoid bloat, I sip rather than drink it—bolting down quantities of ice water at dinner has always struck me as an invitation to instant indigestion. On the other hand, if you are trying to lose weight, savoring a glass or two of water about an hour before meals helps to curb appetite.

3) Do you like fruit? Too much of it, like anything else, is fattening, but when you cut down on the sure fatteners—sugar, pastry, and candy—the natural sweetness of fruit makes an appealing substitute. By this I mean fresh fruit in season.

4) Must you have bread? OK, but have it as the French and the Italians do, without butter at mealtime—there is al-

ready enough butter or oil in the rest of the food. If you are a sandwich fiend, discard the top slice of bread when eating out and make the sandwich open-faced at home. (I assume you use good bread; if it is that sliced white flannel, you might as well throw it out and eat the wrapping.)

5) As you learn to eat less, do you want more taste per ounce, quality rather than quantity? Eliminate highly processed foods. Are you afraid your family might object? Disregard their complaints. Eventually they will come around. (If they do not, let it be known they can market and cook for themselves.)

4

Exit Fat City

Obesity is a form of suicide and, judging by the millions of its practitioners, one of the most popular forms ever devised. I should think an overdose of drugs would be simpler and far less messy, but it appears that efficiency is not the aim in this case. One prefers slow death from an overdose of food.

There is no social stigma attached to overeating. No coroner ever writes that the cause of death was obesity. Your favorite poison is available without prescription at the local grocer's, where, as long as you can pay, no one will ever refuse to serve you. Drink too much at a bar, and you may be bounced. Eat too much at a restaurant, and you become a favorite customer.

You may face job discrimination, especially if you are a woman and expected to be attractive, but few professions will actually exclude you. Of course, you cannot be a jockey, a fashion model, or a dancer, but you can play a role in industry, run a store or a government, or plead a case in court. Even the airlines, while insisting that their flight personnel keep trim, do not dare weigh in passengers along with their baggage, though I think that would be a lovely idea. Why should I pay for thirty pounds of excess baggage when the man next to me does not pay a cent for his fifty pounds of excess flesh?

Mind you, concern about the threat of obesity to health and performance is growing. Unions and municipalities have started to crack down. The Teamsters, for example, have placed a ceiling on fat, and both New York City and Washington, D.C., require policemen to weigh in twice a year. First and foremost, the insurance companies give the obese a hard time. They have been doing it for decades, though I cannot say, looking around me in public, that their strictures have cut much lard.

How could they? Suppose you are penalized or refused a policy—if you have any gumption, you are not going to allow an insurance salesman to tell you how to live. If you thought you would go on forever, you would not, after all, bother with insurance in the first place.

My point is that obesity curtails the pleasure, fun, and adventure of life, as well as shortening life itself. While awaiting all those dreadful, often fatal diseases to which obesity makes you prone, you huff and puff, always short of breath, creak at the joints, suffer from heartburn, hate to undress for sex or beach, and are the brunt of even your closest friends' jokes and supposed jollities, which make you shrivel inside—but not on the surface, where shrinking is needed. There simply are no advantages to being fat. It complicates the most commonplace necessities: using furniture, buying clothes, climbing stairs, passing a turnstile.

(To be morbid, let us list again the maladies more frequent among the obese: arteriosclerosis, arthritis, diabetes, digestive disorders, inflammation of the gallbladder, cirrhosis of the liver, heart disease, hernias of various sorts, high blood pressure, kidney disease, and varicose veins. In fact, of the most common causes of death only tuberculosis and suicide are less frequent in the obese, but, as we have said, obesity is a form of suicide.)

The beautiful people's remedy for obesity is a home brew of preventive medicine, but it is obviously too late for that when you are thirty, fifty, or more pounds overweight. You need someone to take you in hand until you can get yourself under control. You cannot simply eat less, retaining your old habits, because obviously you eat too many wrong foods or you would not be so far gone.

With luck, your case may be diagnosed as middle-aged spread or menopause billow. In other words, you have no past history of serious overweight, but as you hit your prime, you began to sprawl, much to your indignant surprise. After all, you have eaten the same way for years, picking up a few pounds perhaps, but certainly never getting fat. Until now! The case is classic, and the cause is so obvious that it tends to be overlooked. Most of us cannot eat as much after forty as we do at twenty, for the excellent reason that we are less active. Everyone recognizes the former star tackle whose brawn has gone to gut. It does not happen only to athletes out of training; to a lesser degree, it happens to all of us if we do not watch out. We walk less, dance less, play fewer sports, prefer our little comforts, save our energy, fail to cut down on food in proportion—and put on weight. When it comes to women, add the hormonal, and, in some instances, the psychological, upheaval of menopause, and are you really surprised that the scales often go up?

If you do not have a past history of overload—that is, if fat begins at forty-five—chances are that with one concerted effort to reduce you will get back to size and stay there. In other words, after a period of stringent diet, it is a matter of paring down an eating pattern that has become excessive with age, coupled with the rediscovery of the need for regular exercise. Your aim is to retrench, not undertake drastic change.

The plot thickens when a tendency to overweight has been with you all your life. Periodic loss is followed by seemingly inexorable gain until the day you realize you are fifty pounds over and have to reverse the tide. Even more dramatic is that state of addiction and chronic obesity in which you turn to food for consolation as others turn to drugs or drink. Then you need both brainwashing and a kitchen revolution.

In a recent seminar, Dr. George M. Briggs, chariman of the department of nutritional sciences at the University of California, pointed out that "the American public is eating a strange diet. I wouldn't feed it to my cat or dog, let alone to livestock or poultry." Dr. Briggs's prime concern is with malnutrition, but one of the ways that it often shows itself is in obesity. Fat people not only eat too much, they are liable to eat poorly.

Throughout this book, I have given examples of stratagems for eating well and staying thin, and the emphasis has been on do-it-yourself. I do find it absurd for an Austrian princess to enter an expensive clinic to drop eight pounds that she could lose on her own with a minimum of willpower and applied food intelligence. When it comes to fifty pounds, however, going it alone is usually both an illusion and a mistake. You have to be an exception with the self-discipline of a Maria Callas.

"Maria lost an unbelievable amount of weight, and right from the beginning, she started all alone with a little calorie book," says producer and mutual friend Franco Rossellini. "Maria retains water, you see—you must find out why you gain weight. She cannot have salt and has to be very careful with fluids. Now it has become a habit. She always has her calorie book, but mentally she has changed toward food—she has got in the mood, which is what you have to do. Even if she's very thirsty, she would never have a soft drink, because she knows it's bad for her. She would never take three spoonfuls of sugar because she knows they're fattening.

"When we used to work together, she took charge of my diet and would tell me 'No, no, basta!' whenever I went too far, especially with sugar. Do you realize that she had to sue a pasta manufacturer because he claimed she lost weight with his low-cal spaghetti? It wasn't true at all. When I told her I ate pasta, her reaction was violent: 'Never eat pasta, even low-cal; it's terrible for you. The only thing is to use this little book.' Maria is marvelous. She doesn't just count up the calories and then go ahead and eat anything; she's into a permanent diet mood."

Still, Callas is Callas. No doubt she had some professional reasons for slimming down; it allowed her to develop her talent for acting and enhanced her stage presence. On the other hand, she was already world-renowned for her voice, and when you are tops in one field, you usually feel you can damn well afford to be slack in others. How many of us have the discipline (as well as the gift) not only to excel in one endeavor but to make ourselves over as well?

The principal reason for seeking professional help, of course, is to avoid dangerous crash dieting. It is one thing to eat only fruit and yogurt for a week and quite another to cut back drastically on food for a protracted length of time. (You cannot lose thirty pounds overnight, to say nothing of fifty or more.) Any rigid dieting should be carried out under medical supervision, and even if you choose a gradual minimal-weight-loss technique, I think you need to have a doctor check your metabolism and find out whether your fat is associated with other disorders.

In the case of emotional dependence on food, a doctor-mentor to slap your wrist is indispensable; in fact, a daily, rather than weekly, confrontation with Big Brother and the scales would be ideal. As a replacement for the immediate satisfaction of cleaning out the refrigerator, you would have the twenty-four-hour rite of propitiation—pleasing someone whom you respect instead of adding fuel, no matter how luscious, to self-hatred.

The group therapy approach of diet clubs is also a form of psychological control. In addition, competitive spirit is encouraged as members get together weekly to compare weight loss. For some heavies, it works like a charm, and they enjoy the social life such meetings afford. The trouble for others is that everyone is so sympathetic, and you talk so much about eating, that you remain food-oriented. One diet club alumna, a former actress, Doris Konowe, discovered she was in the second category.

"The therapy meeting was like having a sex orgy every week—you were obsessed with it. I lost forty pounds, but I put them back on, in part because you have to measure everything when you're on the club diet. That's a real problem for a compulsive eater. For me it is easier to abstain than to control. And there were no goodies; you weren't allowed any liquor, not even a glass of wine. A lot of people dropped out, they felt so deprived. As far as I could see, the only club people who really succeed are the ones who become group leaders. To qualify, they have to maintain a certain weight." (Needless to say, the leaders are paid, one excellent reason for toeing the line.)

"You know," Doris continues, "they've done tests showing that a fat person can have a meal and, an hour later, eat another. A thin person can't; he feels full and has no appetite. I recall taking lunch to work one day, and a half hour after I'd finished it, a friend said, let's go out to lunch. We got to the restaurant, I ate—and suddenly realized what I'd done."

After trying dozens of diet schemes and giving up on club therapy, she read about Dr. Robert C. Atkins in *Vogue* magazine and has been on his plan with regular checkups ever since. Dr. Atkins is the latest high prophet of high protein (plus low carbohydrate and high fat). He did not invent the concept, and while many doctors do not agree with it, others prescribe similar controversial plans. Sometimes I think that such diets should be embossed with the Stars and Stripes, because high protein is now the All-American way to reduce, and needless to say, the affluent way—quality protein does not come cheap. Such a diet would make me feel ghastly, but then again I do not have fifty pounds to lose and am well aware that there are reasons why you can grow thin on the beasts and fat of the land, the fish that swim, and the birds that fly. (The specific dynamic action of protein, known as SDA, is said to burn up fat more effectively than other nutrients.)

"On the Atkins diet I can indulge in all those marvelous things I'd never been allowed: bacon, cheesecake, whipped cream, nuts—and you can have all kinds of meat," Doris explains. (It worked for her; it may be right for you.)

Is high protein the only way? Of course not. There is a counter school of thought based primarily on cereal grains, vegetables, and fruit, as well as certain dairy products. This approach prevails in Europe and England, but one outstanding American example is Duke University's so-called rice diet (not to be confused with the yin/yang preoccupations of macrobiotics). At Duke you are under constant medical supervision and submit to every test on the books while rice comes out of your ears. However, without the disruption of normal life entailed by booking into a clinic, and by shopping around wherever you live, you are more than likely to find a diet doctor of vegetarian persuasion with whom you can reduce on an outpatient basis. Although I am not a big meat eater, I myself could never be a vegetarian; my choice is a well-balanced diet. The reason I stress alternative, perhaps extremist means for losing weight is that you will not stick out a diet and follow through for maintenance unless you hit on a plan that gives you a kick (and your food kick may be cereal grains). Not only do you need competent supervision, you need a diet you like.

Maybe your temperament is such that you can lick obesity only by having it treated as if it were a rare disease. Take, for example, the Simeons diet, which consists of 500 strictly balanced calories plus one injection per day of human chorionic gonadotrophin, a substance extracted from the urine of pregnant women. According to the late Dr. A. T. W. Simeons, HCG burns up your abnormal fat deposits, which are usually the last to go on diet alone. In other words, with the injections you lose weight where it has accumulated without going scrawny in the face. Many doctors scoff at this idea and attribute the success of the Simeons diet to the placebo effect of the daily checkup and weigh-in. In other words, it is facing Big Brother every day, not the shots, that does it. (The American Medical Association, for one, still considers use of HCG unjustified for weight reduction because of the lack of clinical proof of its effectiveness and safety.)

Nonetheless, this diet, originally developed at the Salvator Mundi International Hospital in Rome, is now used by a limited number of doctors and clinics in the United States, including New York's Kennedy Clinic.

"I think the choice factor in dieting is bad," says television journalist Betty Rollins. "I couldn't possibly cut a little here, a little there; it just doesn't work. I wanted to do something dramatic, and the crazy idea of getting shots appealed to me, especially when I saw that the diet itself wasn't crazy—it wasn't all bananas. Getting shots scared me enough that I didn't dare cheat on the diet. I also felt I had made an investment in money, although the way I did it was not all that costly.

"It's much more expensive at Kennedy Clinic where they prepare the food for you. Instead, I had a nurse give me the shot every day—my own doctor balked. I brought my own 'weighed' lunch to the office, but if I had to eat in a restaurant, it was too embarrassing to carry a postage scale, so I'd have a lobster tail. I don't drink, which meant that not being allowed to didn't bother me. I did discover that eating is a major social habit—after the first week of martyrdom and the second of feeling tired but seeing an improvement, it was the sense of social deprivation, not hunger, that depressed me.

"As far as I'm concerned, it was worth it because I haven't put on any weight since, and I eat normally. For that matter, I eat a lot, though I must say my habits have changed. I totally got over eating sandwiches and rich desserts, maybe out of fear of ever having to go through the cure again. I was so grateful to see an egg when dieting that I think it made me more appreciative of the simple things—I still love to eat a fresh egg. I also find I'm permanently aware of fat and repulsed by it."

Betty had fifteen pounds to lose and shed twelve in the month she went on Simeons. The weight loss is often greater under more highly controlled conditions. You are not allowed to continue for more than a month at a time, the idea being to stabilize at each lower plateau and give the body a rest before renewing treatment. Betty so far has never had to go back and hopefully will never need to. Had she more weight to lose, as do most Simeons patients, she would have signed on for staggered treatments: That's what Patricia Carbine, now of *Ms.* says she has done, and it is what various friends of my friends used to do here in Rome—they would sneak into town, hole up at Salvator Mundi and announce their arrival only when they looked like sylphs.

Instead of injections, intravenous feedings of special formulas, plus strict diet, are the components of the Rossi cure, now popular in Rome, especially among actresses who find it also clears up their skin and makes them feel more limber. After a series of routine tests, from twelve to fifteen feeds are administered at the rate of three a week. The formula varies according to individual need but is always based on sulfurized molecules because of their scavenger qualities. (Other ingredients of the diet cocktail might include triglycerides, thyroxine, and gonadotrophins, which pep you up and make you feel you want to be more active.) The fundamental idea is to detoxify the body, especially the liver. "Obesity is always a form of intoxication," Dr. Rossi says. "The more we eat, the more we have to burn up, and the more waste we accumulate."

During the first week, the patient eats only hulled wheat and apples and may drink black coffee—you will not feel like playing tennis, but you do not have to go to bed. Gradually, potatoes, vegetables, other fruits, and meat are added until individual maintenance level is reached. Weight is lost in spurts, with adjustment intervals in between, because it is felt that losing more than eighteen pounds at a time (roughly one month) is too disrupting to the system.

"Obesity really starts in the head," the doctor explains. "With diet and intravenous feedings, I make sure you lose weight, but all the while I am trying to lower the threshold of appetite, which is determined in the brain. I do it with medicine; someone else might do it with hypnosis. To conquer overweight and obesity, you have to retrain the nervous system—fat is a cerebral condition. Atavistic anxiety makes us all eat more than we need: We may not fear famine but we still believe that one cannot function on an empty stomach. On the contrary, if man wants to save himself, he has to go back to simple food, eat little and only when he's hungry."

Both the Simeons and the Rossi cures sound way out, which may be why they appeal and/or work. Most obese people know they lack common sense about eating, and while waiting for the improbable discovery of some miracle drug to keep them thin without effort, they turn to any new or radical methods. If I were twice my size, I imagine I would not be content to poke along losing a few pounds every month; I would figure that something drastic had to be done. Neither cure, by the way, involves the use of diuretics, nor do other treatments mentioned in this book, because by now most diet specialists have concluded that they induce only temporary weight loss and may aggravate body water changes already out of line in the obese.

As for amphetamines, they have become a rather grim joke in the diet business because of the overgenerous prescriptions of certain New York and London doctors. (Whether or not their patients lost weight, they certainly were flying high, and the higher they flew, the more they wanted, maybe even until they could not get through the day without being drugged.) The usage now, however, is to prescribe amphetaminelike drugs, not for the initial cure, but sparingly during the weight stabilization period.

Many specialists, for example, may advise limited use of amphetaminelike drugs when you have slimmed down but then overindulge and put back a pound or two. The pills help you reinforce your emerging early-warning system in that they suppress appetite until you get it under control. Nonetheless, the advisability of such appetite suppressants remains an open question. A recent study conducted by Dr. Thaddeus Prout of Johns Hopkins for the National Institutes of Health revealed that of ninety-two diet drugs, only one seems to work with no side effects. Need I add that you should never fool around with reducing pills on your own or accept them from well-meaning friends. It's bad enough to be obese without going out of your head.

For heightened perception without drugs plus rapid weight loss, nothing beats the oldest known treatment for obesity: total starvation. Many doctors have turned to the therapy of fasting both to show the patient that considerable weight loss is possible and to utilize the temporary feeling of satiety that occurs when refeeding starts. (Anyone who has ever tried prolonged fasting, whether for spiritual reasons or weight loss, knows that you do not have the time to feel satiated: the first food you turn to tastes so lousy you cannot finish it, and it's easier and better to break a fast with fruit juice or broth.)

I am not talking about a fast or semi-fast once a week or

twice a month, which has become both a chic and perhaps a wise thing to do. I refer, on the contrary, to a fast lasting ten days or more, which is a far more complex undertaking. Because of its association with rites of purification and techniques of social protest, fasting long remained the province of fringe groups: you had to be a crank or a hippie. Even now, the Establishment only recognizes the merit of fasting under carefully controlled conditions. Not everyone can do it.

People suffering from certain illnesses (diabetes, for one) should never be starved, and furthermore, as various tests have shown, fasting produces metabolic changes in any individual that may become irreversible unless they are caught in time. If fasting appeals to you, get your doctor's approval, as well as a referral to a reliable clinic where you will be supervised. Be prepared to feel awful for the first two days, with headache or a funny taste in the mouth, then to feel progressively better. Average weight loss ranges from a pound to two pounds a day, some due to water loss, which does not really count.

In my opinion, the chief result of fasting would be the sudden understanding that you do not need all that food you have been stuffing yourself with. If you can live off your fat for fifteen days and still not be skin and bones, you realize the excess you have been carrying around. This may sound harsh, but true concern about obesity often requires an element of toughness—commiseration gets you nowhere; the only way to help is to prod. With almost no exception, obesity is not fate, bad luck, or a conspiracy of the gods. It is not like a death in the family that throws you for a loop. You alone are responsible; in fact, it is one of the few areas in which you are able to exert total control.

As for the entrenched notions that you have to eat to keep up your strength (even when you are not hungry), or that you cannot function on an empty stomach (even when you are not hungry): get rid of them. It is amazing how little food one needs even in conditions of stress and hyperactivity. I am not suggesting that you use wartime deprivations as a standard or adopt expedition rations as the ideal for city living—by all means benefit from access to a more varied, nutritious diet. Still, you must realize that overeating is not the most exciting thing in life. The following account may help you put your priorities straight.

When Thor Heyerdahl and his crew of volunteers set out on the *Ra* expeditions to prove that an Atlantic crossing was possible in a papyrus-reed craft, they took along much the same food as the early Egyptians might have carried. (This was part of the experiment.) Their basic menu was Egyptian tea or coffee and a piece of bread for breakfast, rice at noon, with more rice for dinner and dried fruit or Moroccan *sello* for dessert. (Because of the humidity, it was safe to cook in the crowded papyrus craft.)

To guarantee safe drinking water, they added tiny pieces of tar to their initial supply of 1,400 liters; as crew member Santiago Genoves, University of Mexico research professor, explains, the use of tar as a water preservative is a Bedouin technique. All the food was stored in terra-cotta jars, including a limited provision of eggs. Again according to ancient practice, they combined 88 percent water and 12 percent cooked lime, placed their eggs in a jar of this milky substance, and forty days later, the eggs were still fresh enough to eat. As for Moroccan *sello*, the *Ra II* staple along with rice, Genoves gives the following ingredients:

wheat flour, 2 kilograms
sugar, 1/2 kilogram
aniseed, 1 kilogram
cinnamon, 100 grams
unflavored gelatin, 1/2 kilogram
sené, 50 grams
butter, 1 1/2 kilograms
honey, 1/2 kilogram

These were roasted and ground to a coffee-colored powder. The ration was one bowl of *sello* to one bowl of water per man, per day.

When the adventurers set off, they joyously hung hams and salami in the cabin and carted on board a three-day supply of tomatoes and fresh fruit (only to discover that combining avocados and *sello* produced explosive diarrhea). Because the crew was international, three kinds of bread were taken: long-lasting Norwegian biscuits, Egyptian bread from an ancient formula, and a Russian hardtack on which one of the crew members broke a tooth in mid-ocean. "Fucking Communist bread," said the victim. "Fucking capitalist teeth" was the Russian's reply. The men had thought to supplement their diet by catching fish (for the protein) and occasionally did, but they were usually too busy, and the Atlantic was either too rough or too polluted. They had a few bottles of wine and champagne—the latter for celebrating when they reached midpoint. The rare treat of wine made them feel awful because their diet was inadequate. Did they lose weight? You bet: an average of 30 percent subcutaneous fat, with the greatest loss among the youngest men.

Now, in order to lose weight, none of you is about to go to sea in a sieve and subsist on rice and Moroccan gruel. But neither will you have the overriding motivation of survival, the intellectual joy of proving a hypothesis, or any sense of freedom and adventure. The *Ra II* mariners, overweight or not, were not in the least concerned about their figures. They accepted not only an unfamiliar diet but also malnutrition as part of the hardship involved in scientific adventure.

One of the major difficulties, I suppose, in losing weight in normal life is that the whole process is such a bore. On the other hand, so is being fat. It is not heroic to stop eating too much; on the contrary, I would say it is common sense, and while the initial phase of stringent dieting takes willpower, once you have redimensioned your attitude toward food, your body will redimension itself. The basic line of attack is not on spare tire, fat bottom, and pot belly; instead you first come to grips with faulty thinking—you get the right amount and the right kind of food on the brain. I have listed various drastic, limited, or tedious reducing techniques more for their shock value than for their practical results. It does not matter how the message gets to the mind as long as it gets there: totting up calories with the satisfaction of Donald Duck's Uncle Scrooge counting his dollars; the drama and suspense of fasting; special injections and intravenous feedings; the total elimination of certain foods for the compensation of eating to satiety on others. . . . Depending on the way your mind functions, you choose whatever convinces you that less is more.

If you are really desperate, you can even turn to the last-ditch therapies of shock treatment or surgery—the latter for reducing specific body areas and the former, as far as I can see, for reducing the brain. Compared with these, hypnosis seems child's play.

I do not know anyone personally who has undergone hypnosis to lose weight, but the idea strikes me as plausible. I do have a friend who tried it to stop smoking.

"I guess I came out from under his spell too soon," she says. "My barely opened eyes caught him ruffling with obvious pleasure through checks and cash on his desk. I don't know why I was so shocked; we all like money, and I must admit he cured me for six months."

One of the most articulate practitioners of hypnotherapy is New York psychiatrist Dr. Abraham Weinberg. He believes that fear of hunger and starvation is atavistic, an overlay of emotional response to food and perhaps inevitable. Food is not just survival. It is fun, comfort, and love. Knowledge of how to prepare and serve it remains one of the more fascinating forms of applied art. Unfortunately, the chronically overweight and obese tend to abuse food, using it to overcome tension, anxiety, depression, or boredom. Unless this attitude is changed, no weight-loss program works for long.

Dr. Weinberg's system includes the basics of a physical checkup and a physician-approved diet and exercise scheme. As he explained when we discussed the problem at length, however, his real goal is to get at the mind: first of all to analyze your feelings about food, and secondly to help you control them. That is where hypnosis comes in, followed by training in autosuggestion.

The patient progresses from sessions with the hypnotist to self-conditioning at home. For example, a half hour before a meal, you lie down, focus eyes upward, then allow your eyelids to close. You count down from ten to one, then take a deep breath and relax. You imagine yourself in divine shape on the diving board, as prima ballerina, or the star of your favorite sex fantasy. Then you switch to a vision of yourself sated from fattening foods, this to be followed by a countervision of your better self enjoying only the right foods. At this point, according to the Weinberg scenario, you can open your eyes and go eat. You feel sufficiently drowsy, relaxed, and psychically stuffed to want very little.

I confess that I could never get through this on my own— either it would give me the giggles or my mind would wander. If you do the cooking, supposedly you can take a half hour between preparing the meal and eating it to unreel this soap opera. Weinberg also advises you to put cotton in your nose to avoid tempting food odors. What about the smell of food burning? I do not do the cooking, but I suspect that most meals cannot be left unmonitored for a half hour while one fantasizes.

As for shock dieting, it is an offshoot of the aversion technique used by psychologists of the behaviorist school to cure a variety of bad habits. So far, its most publicized proponents have been Michael Stokols and Edward Wallach of Miami's Center for Psychological Services. The patient who wants to reduce has a consultation to determine the nature of his compulsive eating. Peanuts, potatoes, doughnuts, ice cream—

whatever it is you cannot resist is offered you in bulk. Electrodes are wired to your hand and for each bite you take, the therapists give you a shock. Furthermore, at initial one-hour sessions, you are not allowed to stop eating. You may even be told just to smell the food and still get shocks.

Each one-hour session costs $35, and for the first months you undertake up to three sessions a week. Some patients are encouraged to continue the treatment at home by acquiring a portable shocker. They either use it on themselves or train someone in the family to give them the jolt. I can assure you that the second time anyone buzzed me, I would throw my plate straight at him, but if you go in for that sort of thrill, who knows? It might work.

As for cosmetic surgery, much as I believe in it for the face —I have had my nose and eyelids done—when it comes to bulging abdomen and thighs, I am still convinced that diet and exercise are the answer. (At most, I believe in body sculpture for the breasts, an area beyond one's control). Nevertheless, if the urge to reform arises when one is already in an advanced stage of belly drag or buttocks spread, recourse to the knife may give such encouraging, quick results that one determines to stay in shape forever after. Particularly with women who are heavy only from the hips down, the temptation must be strong to lop off what seems to be one of Nature's bad jokes.

Various U.S. specialists remain skeptical about the results of body sculpture. First of all, they think there is too much scarring, and secondly, woe betide you if you go back to your former gluttony and split your new seams. For that matter, watch out you do not get back into circulation too soon. A very chic French friend of mine was so proud of her new body and so eager to show it off back home that her seams split on the airplane.

On the other hand, my good friend Brazilian plastic surgeon Ivo Pitanguy, routinely turns out new bottoms and bellies and finds it gives most clients a new lease on life—or at least puts them back on the beach.

His complex technique for abdominal reduction makes the final suture a narrow scar almost level with the pubic hair line, which means a bikini would cover it. My first reaction to this is that if you are so thick in the middle that you need surgery, you are probably too old and much too big all over to wear a bikini. That by no means implies you should not go swimming—one-piece bathing suits exist.

On the other hand, I have not had five pregnancies, any Caesareans, or other abdominal operations. For a woman in basically good shape who justifiably cannot pull in the slack of life, abdominal surgery makes sense. As it is, when an obese patient has an appendectomy, for example, it is rather common surgical practice to remove impedimental fat. There are no aesthetic motives in mind—the surgeon merely removes any fat (usually a very small amount) that gets in the way of his doing his job. No sense asking him to take out more; he would refuse. The plastic surgeon's aim, on the contrary, is a flat belly, so he takes out what he can without disturbing vital organs.

As for advanced buttocks spread, when other treatment fails or seems worse than surgery you might as well have it sliced off. In about ten days, you can sit down again. Ideally, all that remains is a bit of hand stitching under the gluteal fold.

The last hope—the light at the end of the tunnel of obesity —is the intestinal bypass operation. The operation consists of severing the small intestine near the end of the jejunum, then reconnecting it just above the beginning of the colon. This shortens the length of the active small intestine from twenty-three feet to about thirty inches. Food passes through the system quicker, and caloric absorption is reduced. In consequence, a person should stop gaining and supposedly even lose weight without having to diet. Reportedly one patient found that after the operation she developed an inexplicable craving to eat mud, but her reaction seems to be unique. Needless to say, it is the general consensus among doctors that the bypass operation should be performed only in rare cases.

Personally, I do not believe in crash methods, however fat you may have become over the course of the years. I may be wrong, and the effortless, miracle solution to obesity could be right around the corner. With many pounds to lose, I would certainly go to a doctor, but I would prefer someone like London's Dr. Mary Austin, a homeopath and one of the most consulted Western practitioners of acupuncture, who tries first of all to make you think.

"I start by asking patients whether they know how big their stomach is," she says. "They never know, so I get them to join both hands in front of the body with all fingers touching. Then they are told to open their hands as if cupping water with the fingertips still touching, except for the thumbs. That is the size of your stomach, I explain, and if you fill that three times a day, you are overeating.

"I make you feel as ashamed as possible. If you put in rubbish, of course, you get a rubbishy body. I advise keeping food and drink separate; it is all right to sip with meals, but pushing down food with liquids only makes you blow up. Each patient is told to eat flesh, vegetables, and fruit with a big draft of Adam's ale midmorning and afternoon—Adam's ale is water—to help you throw off toxins. You should be a river, not a pond. Then we decide what else a patient can eat, or not, according to character, medical history, age, and flesh group.

"After three weeks, I see how the patient adjusts mentally. If he hasn't the sense to see what we're driving at, if he is too stupid, then I work out a specific list of don'ts. I'd rather not have to bother. After a while, should any illness lurking behind obesity rear its head, I treat it. Often the dieting itself cures the problem.

"You should never go onto a diet too fast—they don't pour the blood into you when you have a transfusion; it goes in drop by drop so you can take it. The quicker you lose a lot of weight, the quicker you put it back on. I am sick of hearing about diet fads. Food today is colossally varied, and that's what you have to learn to cope with. But you have to do it at your level. We are individuals."

5

Weighing In at the Fat Farm

The French, the Italians, and the Germans have always had their spas; the Swiss, their mountain air retreats. The Americans pioneered in beauty resorts, and the English developed the naturopathic country manor. Put them all together and they spell fat farms. It is amazing how many people have been to them. Some even go back.

The idea is that you sign in, preferably for two weeks or a month, and the farmhands—doctors, therapists, yogis, nutritionists, and beauticians—pull together what you have let go. At the end of your stay, you have lost weight and toned muscles. Your skin is clearer and less slack, and you have probably discovered that relentless exposure even to brown bread and raw vegetables, honey and fruit can be too much of a good thing.

In England there are about fifteen health hydros to choose

from. In the United States, in addition to the well-established luxury beauty farms such as Elizabeth Arden's two Maine Chances (one in Arizona), California's Golden Door, and the Texas Greenhouse, several dozen new health spas have sprouted. Some are combination resort-spas (Rancho La Puerta and La Costa near San Diego, for example), others are austere establishments devoted to health through fasting (Dr. Shelton's in Texas, Esser's Ranch in Florida, and Pawling Manor in New York). According to a recent American Hotel and Motel Association listing, hotels and motels in thirty-seven American cities now offer spa facilities. In some cases, this boils down to a small swimming pool and the odd steam cabinet; in others, it means a substantial array of reducing machinery but no medically controlled diet plan. If you are going to a fat farm for more than the briefest stay, it is wise to inquire carefully about facilities and diet.

The American luxury farms do get surprisingly fast results. Cristina Ford was confounded by the Arizona Maine Chance, where she went once out of curiosity. She happens to have a marvelous figure, so it was not a miracle that she emerged in top shape. Still, it is gratifying (at more than a hundred dollars a day) to see that they know their business.

"I flew from the beauty farm to Washington to attend a party with former President Johnson," Cristina says. "As I was dressing, I got on the scale and realized that, instead of losing weight, I had gained a pound—mind you, the diets there are vegetarian, so I ate their non-diet food, which is permitted. But that's not the point. My dresses were falling off me; my slacks wouldn't stay up. An additional pound means nothing when your waistline suddenly looks like the stem of a wine-glass. Five hours of gym and one hour of swimming per day had made me taut."

Vera Maxwell keeps a small painting done by Prince Rainier in the living room of her New York apartment. Three fat ladies walk toward a green house in the middle of the painting. On the other side of the house the same three ladies, nude, light as air, are flying on angel wings. The prince gave it to the designer as a souvenir of the two-week cure she took with Princess Grace and her sister at Neiman-Marcus's Greenhouse in Dallas, Texas.

"I think we both lost more inches than pounds—I lost only four pounds," says Mrs. Maxwell. "I remember Fleur Cowles was there, and the first night Grace and I were so starved we ate the parsley off her plate. We still had hunger pains the second night, not realizing that you could call down and have skimmed milk sent up.

"You soon get used to it. We were on neither maintenance nor minimum diet; we had 1,000 calories per day, and the food—what there was of it—was marvelous. We had fish and meat only twice a week, but there were endless, beautiful soufflés (made with broccoli or lobster or apricot and using one yolk to three egg whites).

"The reason you lose inches is that they work you from dawn to dusk. It's 'wake up and shine' at 8:30 with a series of different exercises, including 'swing and sway' to music. Later, half the group has its toenails done while the rest are in the pool for water exercise—they say at the clinic that movement in water puts less strain on the heart than 'dry' calisthenics.

"The only thing we really didn't like was that we couldn't find a place to take a walk. Despite all the exercise, you long to get out for a quiet stroll. In Texas, they've got nothing but roads with cars coming at you. Grace and I gave up—the closest we came to nature was getting stuck on the sandy 'soft shoulders' on the side of a road."

Actor Van Johnson had a quite different experience. He told me that during one of his stays in England he slipped off to Enton Hall to try to drop a few pounds.

"I'd been living at the Connaught," he said, "and you know the groceries there. The clinic looked like something out of an Alec Guinness movie, as though everyone had come there to die. First, they explained that you have to start from the insides out. That's nothing new—talk to Gloria Swanson, she's an enema baby, and Mae West is the queen of colonics. I wasn't allowed in the dining room for ten days, and it worked. I lost fourteen pounds. That English circuit is incredible—there's another clinic called Forest Mere. All I can say is, better Forest Mere than Forest Lawn."

At present, more and more Americans are trying the English hydros. They combine the cure with a holiday or a business trip abroad, taking advantage of the lower cost for slimming (about $25 to $35 a day). Cappy Badrutt once tried a long weekend with actress Joan Collins at Buxted Park.

"It was a very mixed crowd," she said. "You exercised with enormously fat people. There were hot pools to stand in, cold water to jump in and out of, boys and girls together, and the usual saunas and cabinets. Every hour was filled, and when they did allow you a free moment, you were expected to go out and breathe the fresh air.

"We laughed like mad at the very idea that we had paid to put up with this. First they lined you up like soldiers and then, around late afternoon, they killed you off—and it wasn't with kindness. After a jaw-binding supper of grass salad and nuts, we would spend the evening limply watching TV. In all fairness, I must say I lost five pounds in three days and looked ten years younger."

Buxted Park is no more. Toward the end (after Cappy's time), it was surely worth the trip—and, from what I'm told, for more than losing weight: helicopters disgorging the fat rich on the lawn, Rolls-Royces in the driveway, parties of gays out from London, older men with pretty young things, champagne in the bedrooms, first-rate massage and treatment. "My dear, it became a whorehouse," sniffed one austere fat farm devotee. Buxted is no more because a sheik from the Trucial States liked it so much that he bought it.

"You must realize that life has changed in the sheiks' harems," says journalist Eve Arnold, who did some memorable reportage on the cloistered ladies. "They are making the women slim down because they weren't living long enough and grew old before their time. Inside the harem, those fantastic masks and veils come off, you know. The ladies now read *Vogue* and take the Pill."

At latest report, no harem ladies are being slimmed at Buxted, but a neighboring gardener says that the sheik is certainly not neglecting the grounds. They have never looked better.

Eve, who is London-based, even tried a fat farm herself— a weekend at Forest Mere. If she does a book this year, she plans to go straight to a farm to work on it, not for the diet, but because it is like living in a womb—a cocoon of care.

"I lost five pounds in four days, and I felt marvelous afterward," she explains. "There's a good pub in the nearby village. All the men at the farm would sneak out at night like errant children and hold up in the back room, then sweat it off the following day. (Men lose water more easily.) They had to lock the fridge at the farm or they would find starving people wandering around in the middle of the night on a pantry raid.

"But the service is fantastic. They used to tuck me in between electric blankets—I was just floating. I had this tremendous feeling that people really cared. It gives you a sense of well-being."

This one can understand. Overweight or not, who does not love and need to be pampered and clucked over once in a while? Wives or husbands, lovers, and friends cannot always do it—they may need the treatment themselves. If you have children, they often demand rather than give loving attention, and rightly so. The clinics' outstanding attraction probably is that they fulfill the role of ersatz mother, attentive, yet wisely severe, and provide a climate that encourages you to shape up and do something. The emotionally stable purr when pampered. How much more it must help those obese who eat because they are affection-starved.

At the Metropole Hydro in Brighton, the emotions that underlie poor physical condition and fat are explored by means of a color test. The test, based on eight colors, of which blue, green, red, and yellow are the most important, was devised by Dr. Max Luscher, professor of psychology at Basle University, as a means of determining psychological disposition. You are asked to look at a number of panels, each with a selection of different colors or different hues of the same color. Without stopping to think, you pick from each panel the color you like best, then second, third, on down to the one you like least. You are made to move fast to avoid choosing through association with fashion, furnishings, or art, which most people tend to do if given time to reflect.

Mrs. Jo Scott, who does the testing at Brighton, worked with it previously at another English fat farm. Her experience confirms the findings of Swiss researcher Helmut Klar that obese women, when tested, show a marked preference for blue, followed by green, both passive colors. At the same time they object to the active colors red and yellow. On the Luscher scale, blue (particularly the dark blue of the night sky) is not only the color of quiescence, it is also associated physiologically with sweetness. In other words the blue ladies craved love, but were probably thwarting their desire by eating sweet things and getting fat instead. Supposedly, color preference swings with shifts in weight, though this is hard to prove.

Along with the extra fillip of the test, the Metropole—in contrast to most English hydros, which are usually buried at the bottom of countryside and garden—also affords a view of the sea, to say nothing of Brighton Pier and the hordes who come down from London when the weather is good. I mention this because in choosing a clinic the location is important.

The sea either unnerves or braces you, the mountains obsess or exhilarate, the country depresses or calms. You go where you know you feel good to begin with.

Anne-Marie Bennstrom, who runs The Sanctuary in Los Angeles and Hollywood, is convinced that the right environment is essential. At her Los Angeles spa out-of-towners can live in while locals trim on a daily/weekly basis. The right environment, on her terms, is sun, air, and water. In addition, "to lose weight," she says, "you live like an ancient Buddhist: you fast, you walk, and you rest." No matter that she learned about fasting and organics in the jungle in Guatemala, the principle holds.

I have never been to a fat farm to lose weight, partly because of temperament and partly because I live in Italy, where they do not exist. Our spas, though they have begun to cater to slimming and beauty, are still more interested in aching bones, ailing livers and kidneys, and the erections and ovaries that fail. This is glossed over with a smattering of culture. At Montecatini, in particular, you cannot fail to notice from the assorted photographs and plaques that Verdi, Mascagni, Puccini, and other greats of Italian opera were the spa freaks of their time. You still get music, either live or canned, in the pavilions where you take the waters. The music counterpoints the flushing of thousands of toilets as the waters take hold.

From what I hear, a stay at a spa or fat farm elsewhere can also be a shattering experience. On the one hand, the Cecil B. DeMille approach, common to many American clinics, is enough to make you think that a few extra pounds, if gained over good food, talk, and wine, are part of what living is all about—a hallmark of civilization. All those pseudo-Roman baths, prana salads, Aztec vapors, pink sweatsuits, jogging tracks on manicured lawns, and herbal swaddlings soon make you feel that you, and everyone else in the place, are made of plastic.

On the other hand, the enforced gentility of some of the

English farms barely conceals an underlying madness. As a London businessman confessed, comparing notes on high colonics and the wheel of life over boring food was so grim that it sent him straight back to the bottle he was supposed to be drying out from. Mystic experience drove another London acquaintance back to city stress in a hurry. "The owner of this spa was really trying for levitation—it was the most awful atmosphere, and that music temple with the sunken organ didn't help. In class, we were all to close eyes and hold hands. One lady squeezed mine, and I instantly disconnected left and right. I believe evil can be passed as well as good, if anything can. The owner would try laying of hands on you while you were lying there. I saw girls in screaming hysterics."

To some extent, I imagine that fat farms are always pot luck. You never know who you will find next to you, nude or clutching a towel, in hydrotherapeutic togetherness. The amenities, especially in England, vary with the seasons. In February you are liable to discover that the heated pool listed in the brochure is covered with snow—they heat it for summer use. Again, the answer is to find out all you can about the setup before you check in. Prices vary in every country and do not always correspond to accommodation, which may range from spartan through the latest in modern convenience to the rare, old-fashioned luxury of manor house with rolling grounds. Most clinics are vegetarian, though not all of them are adamant about it. Be wary of any descriptions of a so-called average day. In serious clinics programs are modified according to individual need and you and your neighbor may have a quite different average day at the same spa.

Nevertheless, in general the beauty farms are designed to put you through at least four hours a day of land and/or water exercise. Usually the huff and puff starts very early in the morning and while on the first day this is grim to anyone out of training, the second reveille is murder. (Every bone creaks, every muscle aches, and you are convinced that if you get out of bed, you will have a heart attack.) Strenuous exercise is interspersed with massage, herbal wraps, and baths, as well as the relief of sybaritic beauty treatments.

On the other hand, at health clinics where you can fast, strenuous exercise and beauty care are minimal, with the emphasis instead on hydrotherapy, leisurely walks, and rest. When deciding where you will go, it helps to bear this basic divergence in mind. Thus whether or not you are completely pleased once you are at your chosen spa, at least you will have chosen one that is somewhat close—in that it's either active or passive—to what you were looking for.

"A hydro is not the same as a beauty farm, that I can tell you," says a journalist friend. "Unless you are ready for the old folks' home, forget any place like Shrubland Hall, especially in the winter. I knew the gardens and grounds, which are superb, would be dormant, but indoors was even more so —starving patients were falling asleep in their armchairs.

"The decor was very 'gracious living': a staircased entrance of exquisite proportion, lots of books to read, a display of fine porcelain, and handsome sitting rooms. If you like plants—I do—there was even one of the incredible northern conservatory rooms where you freeze but greenery thrives. Nothing institutional about our Shrubland, that's for sure, except for the soup at noon and the clammy treatment rooms in the basement. Have you ever had a sitz bath? Don't try it in a dungeon.

"There was no exercise program, only an average of two treatments per day, hydro or mild massage. Winter sports consisted of Scrabble and stomach rumblings. Constipation was the rule. One soon discovered that the line formed to the right outside the infirmary where pills were dispensed. Inmates referred to them as the brown bombers. So much for gracious living!

"The whole establishment was geared to an invalid's pace, and, unsurprisingly, the happiest patients were those who loved to drowse because they were fasting—progressing from lemon-honey-water to the raptures of potassium broth and fruit juice. Apparently, after abstinence, your first go at potassium freaks you out. There were girls who could not sleep at night. A rotund Latin American was enchanted with his stay. In five weeks he had lost almost forty-two pounds. I would have lost my mind. Believe it or not, I discovered that many peoply fly to a fat farm every year; it's become part of their life-style."

People with weight problems do become addicted to the cure. When the seasons change, they automatically migrate to one of the farms to bolster themselves for the long, hard winter, or even more crucial as the years go by, to shape themselves up for the sun. The biennial weighing-in would not be enough in the case of obesity, but I think, if you enjoy it, such a plan can solve minor overweight problems, and you enjoy the side benefits of exercise, rest, and beauty care. Instead of coming back from weekend trips and vacations fatter and more tired than you were before, you come back from clinic vacations thinner and more relaxed—at least for a while. For almost anyone, it is strangely soothing to watch the animal perform, get the skin and toenails sparkling, and pull in the slack.

Both Princess Ira Furstenberg and Alba, hairdresser to the chic in Rome, are habituées of the Swiss Valmont, one of the best diet clinics, though not a beauty farm in the usual sense of the word. Valmont's specialty is custom-made diets. It is not vegetarian, though an apples-only cure is recommended. Ira and Alba go there regularly because they find it just like any first-rate Swiss hotel—"how divine to find impeccable service in the middle of the woods with a lake." The added bonus is that you come away thin.

London's beautiful Pat Harmsworth believes in slipping away to a health farm for a concentrated effort a couple of times a year. She often does a semifast on her own during weekends at the family house in the country, but that is not the same as having a real go.

American Lois Sieff, married to the owner of Marks & Spencer, says that she has been to a dozen places and intends to keep going back. Her husband, whose nutritional convictions tend toward porridge and other rib-stickers, teases her that she must not get too thin. She is not thin; she is fine.

"If you really want to know how I keep my 'gorgeous figure,'" she says laughing, "come over for lunch, and we'll talk about it." Her system is knowing she needs one. "Once or twice a year, I go to a clinic," she explains. "The results hold about three months, then start going phlooey. I check in just before I'm back where I started."

Fashion designer Bill Blass, who goes twice a year to the Golden Door, is also a clinic enthusiast. "Going to a farm has saved my life."

Removed from jet-set pressures but subjected to plenty of others, the dean of a New England women's college makes a point of slipping away once a year to a New Jersey spa to be hounded, pounded, and pampered. (As a regular routine, she runs two miles along the Charles River three times a week.)

These are people with high standards who are basically in good shape—the clinics have only to slim them down a bit and tone them up. The case of the chronically fat person who decides to try a farm because home remedies have not worked is quite different.

Fat farms have no reliable statistics on how many customers keep off the weight they lost at the clinics. For many whose eating pattern is obviously wrong—or they would not be obese to begin with—the recommended follow-up diets are too foreign to their normal eating habits. The stomach has "shrunk," but the mind balks, and with no one to slap their wrists, the fat rolls on again.

The advantage, and eventual shortcoming, of the farms is that every day is planned and every move monitored. You are kept away from food. For consolation, there is the knowledge that everyone else in the place is suffering too; it becomes a form of group therapy. Unfortunately, you tolerate the routine only because it is brief, like doing your hitch in the army reserve.

Instead of taking food off your mind, clinic life seems to put it on the brain, even when you are not hungry. From the moment you strike up a conversation with a fellow patient, all you ever talk about is eating: the last great meal, the five best ways to do truffles, your favorite candy bar, recipes for pork pies. . . . In the States you play the ice cream game: how many flavors can you remember?

Still, even if you are obese and not just seasonally overweight, the clinics may be the first step in the right direction. If nothing else, they will force you to lose enough pounds or inches to show that it can be done. In the initial stage, removal from professional or home pressures can be crucial. (A young housewife phones her husband from a fat farm to tell him that she has lost two inches off her thighs. "And seven off your bust?" he inquires. That is a supportive husband for you—just try to diet with someone like that around!)

There are other psychological weight deterrents in clinic life that I would find effective, whether or not they are inadvertent. One is the depressing, isolated atmosphere—many of the farms achieve this effect to a stunning degree. You leave them thinking you would do anything rather than have to go back again. In addition, the jazziest American farm and most of its low-keyed English cousins share an ultimate weapon—the sight of all that fat in the communal saunas, the echoing sound in the massage department of acres of flesh being slapped about. Are they moving mountains? Just about. This in itself should put you off sugar and starch forever.

My mother picked up some of her frugal food habits years ago when she went to the vegetarian Bircher-Benner clinic near Zurich. The late Dr. Max Bircher-Benner, who opened his first establishment at the turn of the century, was one of the earliest advocates of nutritional therapy based on raw foods. This was before vitamins had been heard of, much less become an obsession.

The clinic is now supervised by his niece, Dr. Dagmar Lichtie, who has been described as "a fabulous woman who goes to India once a year and has a sign in her office to the effect that health is not the absence of disease; it is a complete sense of well-being." Bircher-Benner is definitely a health farm—no fun and games in pink sweatsuits here. Special regimens are available for poor circulation, high blood pressure, arteriosclerosis, liver problems, rheumatism, and so on, as well as for obesity. In addition to diet, cures usually include hydrotherapy, breathing exercises, dry brushing, early morning walks, sun baths, and light baths. Meals are not limited exclusively to raw foods; however, it is a basic tenet that all meals should start with them.

"The food is unbelievably good, at least to my taste," says Emilio Pucci, who goes there for three or four days once a year. "In the morning you have fresh fruit, Bircher-muesli, rose-hip tea with brown sugar, whole wheat bread and butter. For lunch you might have wheat-germ cutlets with cranberry juice and their raw vegetables, which are absolutely divine.

"The last time I went there, I arrived on a Monday in a state of complete mental and physical exhaustion. It was a little over a month since I had broken a vertebra and had twenty-four stitches after a ski accident. I flew from Hawaii, where I had gone on a business trip, to Rome, drove to Florence, and then to Zurich. When I left the clinic the following Friday, I felt on top of the world. It's true they give you a thorough checkup. It's also true that I don't drink and I don't smoke, so I pick up fast, but that still doesn't explain it. Often, after the first day and a half at the clinic, I've experienced terrible pain in the legs, then it goes away. They say it's the toxins in the muscle—we are all poisoned either by wrong food or by nervous stress. Their aim is to disintoxicate and restore balance."

Pucci, who is impeccably lean and straight, does not go to Bircher-Benner to lose weight. He goes to unwind and start ticking again. On the contrary, when my mother went, she wanted to slim. Many clients combine the two.

Without making a cult of the clinic's famous "muesli" (a blend of oats, condensed milk, lemon juice, shredded apple, and nuts), and without abandoning meat or pasta altogether, my mother permanently adopted two clinic principles, one radical and the other as obvious as the fact that we all speak prose. The radical notion was that you feel better if you eat less. As for the obvious, she simply reinforced a natural Italian liking for salads and raw fruits. She might eventually have come upon this herself; the fact is that the clinic converted her earlier.

I think my mother was right. You go to a clinic with an open mind, just as you might try anything new to see what it has to offer. You adopt what is good for you and what you enjoy enough to stick with. If you discover—as she did not—that periodic stays at a farm are the easiest way for you to remain slender and keep in top condition, you organize your schedule accordingly. I would never do that. I do not have the time and prefer to spend my money on greater pleasures, but I confess that I would adore to try a farm once and get the works—four or five days devoted entirely to the body beautiful. I think it would be great fun and good for the morale.

English actress and pop star Jane Birkin packed off to a farm once with her father and her baby girl. She had just split up with her husband and felt herself unraveling.

"I was in a huge crisis and couldn't have picked a better place. You have to get up at seven for gym and face the myna bird. We shrieked out the exercise count with the instructress. You staggered wearily through the day with everything designed for pain, especially the massage machines. I also remember I felt quite hungry. But going there was great for me because I laughed so much. The people were so strange. By early evening everyone who was banned from the dining room went to bed. We used to walk down to feed the ducks.''

In Jane's case, I know her stay was good for the morale. She sent her estranged husband the bill.

6

Eating Out Is Not Overeating

Traveling, dining out, entertaining—no doubt about it, that is when restraint and diet are cast to the winds and, to my mind, rightly so.

It is not the occasional splurge that does you in; it is over-consuming *all* the time. If your regular eating pattern keeps your weight in line, I say join the party. There are ways to splurge without incurring disaster on the scales. The idea is to indulge yourself rarely, only by choice, and to compensate quickly. I, for instance, am invited out about five times a week. I have a food orgy about twice a month.

By food orgy I do not mean twelve courses and five hours at table, which strikes me as a bore. I mean a beautiful meal with just enough of the wrong things to eat and drink to make it right and give you that luscious stuffed feeling. What I do avoid and find revolting is overeating just because of circumstances, when it is no fun and you really do not want to.

To take traveling first, the parody of the gourmet life is the business trip. At every stop you are wined and dined as if it were crass to get on with the matter at hand without first being stuffed like a pig. What started as a courteous, propitiatory rite has become a drag—if not a major contributory cause of heart attack—for everyone concerned, whether visiting firemen or hosts on home ground. If we could go back to passing the peace pipe, instead of the double martinis and triple portions, before making our business deals, we would be much better off. As it is, the only sensible course is to concentrate on the fare that is least fattening and most digestible, pick at the rest, and try to arrange a few quiet mealtimes for yourself. The other trick—and this applies to any sort of air travel—is to rest rather than eat on planes, where the food, however glowingly described, has all the zest of "early cardboard" TV dinners.

I do not know why the business world and the planners of other official trips remain so retrograde in their food thinking. Everyone knows that a business trip or a diplomatic mission is not a fiesta. They have learned to consider the time lag. What about a food lag? Queen Elizabeth II, with a sovereign's prerogative, asked on her last trip to France that the food be kept simple: two courses and a pudding would be lovely. The French were scandalized. But no matter what you think of pudding—maybe not much—the queen's approach was absolutely right.

When I do promotion tours in the United States, my eating gets down to a formula. For breakfast I have tea, as usual, plus an egg. If I have to grab a fast lunch out between appearances, I do not expect the mozzarella and tomato I would have in Rome. I order a hamburger with French fries, push off the bun, scrape aside the potatoes (they have to be there so I can snitch five with my fingers), and concentrate on the meat. No soft drink, no milkshake. If I am still hungry, thank God for cottage cheese!

When I have a business appointment for lunch, I resign myself to richer food, knowing both that it is bad for me and that I cannot resist it entirely. In New York, at the beginning or end of a tour, when someone says, "Let's have a bullshot," I have one; nor, before it closed, could I ever pass up the crêpes with sauce at Le Pavillon. Needless to say, while on tour, with a sixteen-hour-a-day work schedule, I never touch alcohol. I could not take it. At night, no matter what the city, restaurant, or company, I keep dinner simple. I have a steak, one of those fabulous baked potatoes, and a salad.

After trips to the States, I always yearn for raw foods, but when you travel on business, you have to learn to adapt to what is readily available. At least I avoid most packaged, canned, and frozen produce.

Usually, I can also arrange to keep a few lunch- and dinner-times to myself. I find a minute during the day to buy dried apricots, yogurt, a piece of roast chicken, and a tomato and then slip them into my hotel room. Or I ask room service for the freshest fruit and salad they can muster. Sometimes I even skip dinner and go to bed early with bottled water and fruit juice. The irony is that beautiful fruit and salads are plentiful in the States. Why is it that in restaurants they are all jazzed up, the fresh fruit chopped and mixed with frozen or canned fillers and the salad tossed with bottled dressings and other extraneous matter such as croutons, hunks of stale cheese, and garlic? Whatever happened to plain salad vinaigrette?

Sometimes I can work in a weekend or a Sunday with American friends at their home. Then I eat very well: fresh produce and simple food. It is the constant socializing in restaurants that is the pitfall when on tour. If I did not watch myself, I would put on twenty pounds.

Happily, traveling on your own is quite different. You are free to pace yourself, including your own dining preferences. An important part of the trip may be the leisurely memorable meals. But do you really want memorable meals twice a day?

I should think not. Those meals will have greater significance and less devastating consequences if they are interspersed with regular light, sensible meals.

Most Americans find they put on weight in Europe. They are not used to all that food, good or bad, especially the heavy lunches. Most Europeans traveling in the United States find that they put on weight there. They attribute it to the fabulous sandwiches, ice cream, milkshakes, and cocktails, none of which are gourmet but all of which delight them. In both cases the problem is probably that customary eating habits are combining forces with a hunger born of curiosity. The American abroad still wants his big breakfast as well as a European lunch and his drinks and snacks. The European counts on his regular courses and something mildly alcoholic to drink with them, then adds American desserts and snacks.

Also, when traveling you eat out most of the time and feel that in strange restaurants you cannot order just a few light things that may be all you want. There is something about going to a restaurant that in itself induces overconsumption. Again, this is marvelous if you go there on purpose because the food is good, and you compensate for the indulgence by eating less before and after. On the other hand, when you are surfeited and longing for just a light meal, the answer is: order it. Just because the custom calls for various courses, you are not obliged to have them. Ten years ago, even five, European waiters may have sneered. Not anymore! Their regular clientele, whom they count on during the long off-tourist season, has grown more weight-conscious and changed all that.

Another system friends of mine use when traveling is selective eating by country. In Britain they take advantage of the wonderful large breakfasts and delicious teas; in Paris they hit the croissants, red meat, cheese, and wine; and in Italy, more wine but with pasta, field salad, artichokes, and fruit. Whether or not it all balances out, the idea is to concentrate on the special, local delights you cannot resist and play down the rest.

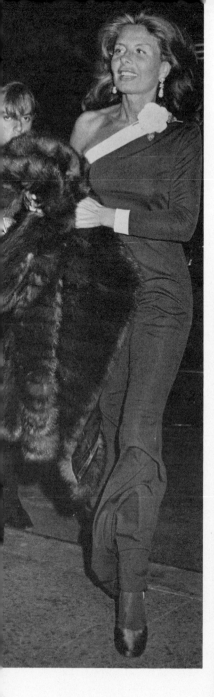

Cristina Ford, here arriving at New York's "21" Club, is a "true believer" who does daily calisthenics and takes three-mile walks. (*Women's Wear Daily*)

Former model Betsy Theodoracopulos substitutes conversation for hors d'oeuvres at Giorgio Sant'Angelo's cocktail party. (*Women's Wear Daily*)

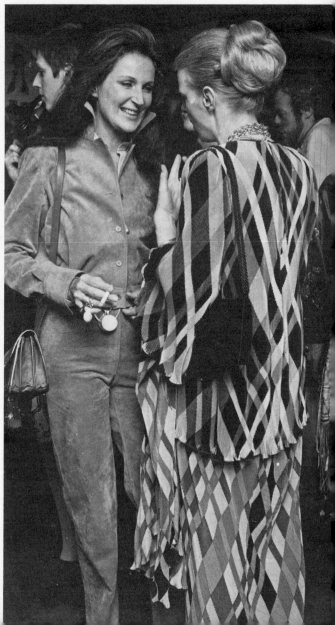

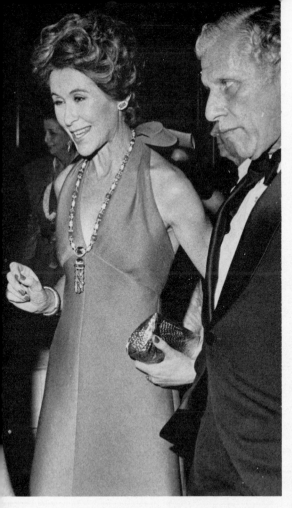

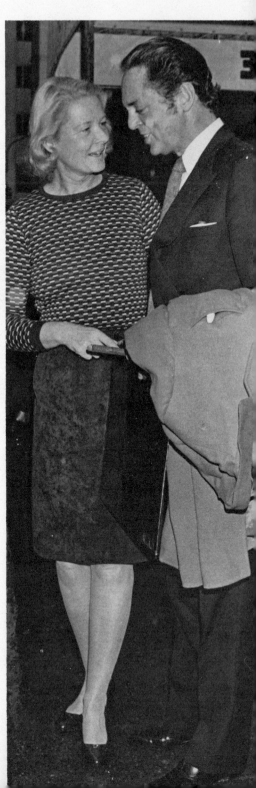

Anyone can clearly see that Betsy Bloomingdale, partygoing at El Morocco, is a believer in the body beautiful. (*Women's Wear Daily*)

You can bet that Ceezee Guest and Baron Alexis de Rede ate sparingly during an informal luncheon at La Grenouille in New York. (*Women's Wear Daily*)

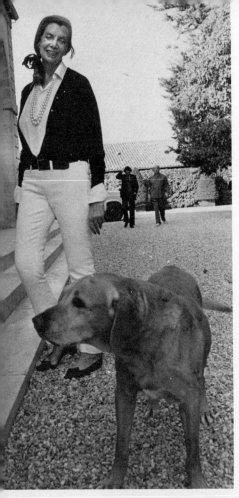

Baroness Pauline de Rothschild returns to the famous Château Lafite-Rothschild after her morning constitutional. (*Women's Wear Daily*)

At a theater opening in New York, champagne glass in hand, Arlene Dahl would argue that occasional splurges are good for the soul. (*Women's Wear Daily*)

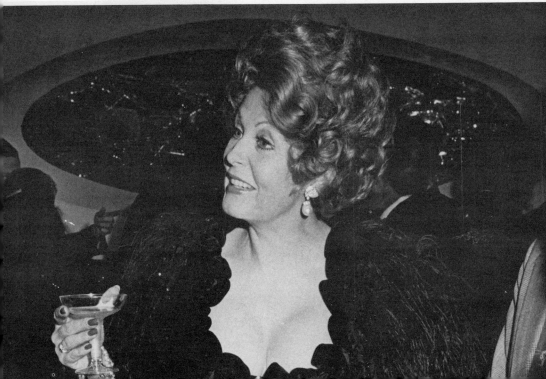

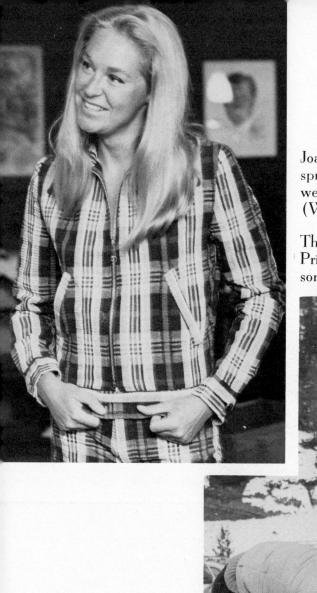

Joan Kennedy on a casual shopping spree in New York; if you're going to wear jeans, you'd better look like this. (*Women's Wear Daily*)

The whole family should exercise! Here Princess Ira von Furstenberg and her son ski in the Dolomite Alps. (ANSA)

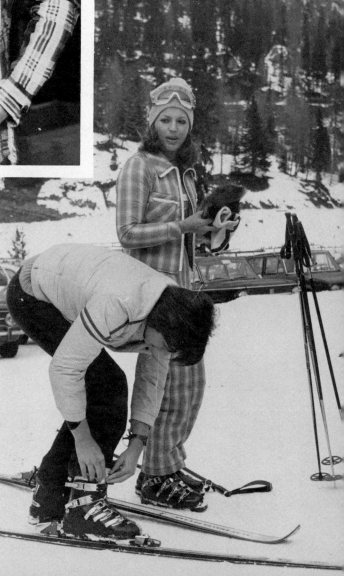

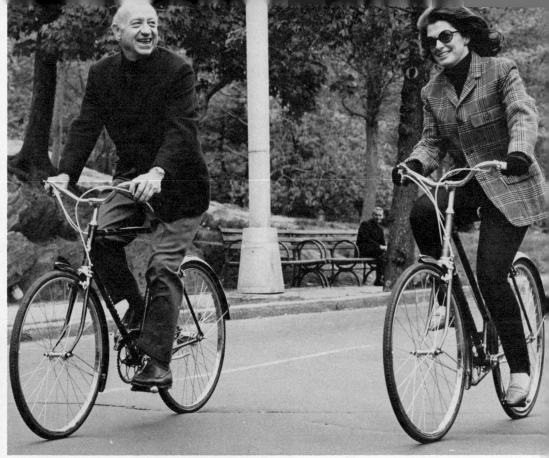

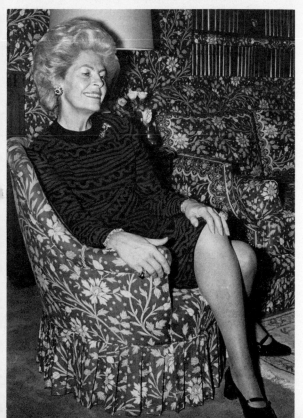

Senator Jacob Javits and his wife, Marion, keep in shape with frequent bicycle rides in Central Park. (UPI)

Relaxing at home in Paris after many state dinners and receptions, Mme Nicole Alphand practices what she preaches about dieting. (*Women's Wear Daily*)

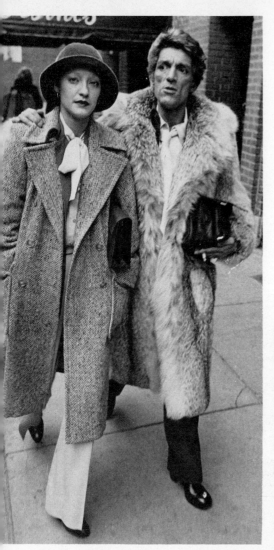

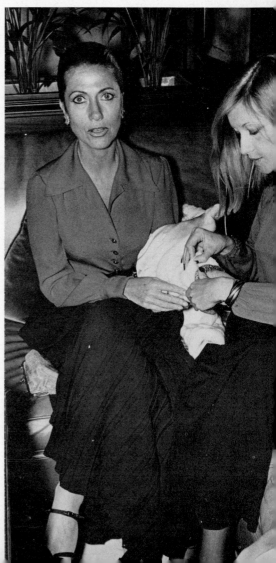

Loulou de la Falaise and Giorgio Sant'Angelo take a brisk stroll after lunching at Orsini's in New York. (*Women's Wear Daily*)

Taking a break from her busy work schedule, Hélène Rochas has won the struggle to resist overeating at business lunches. (*Women's Wear Daily*)

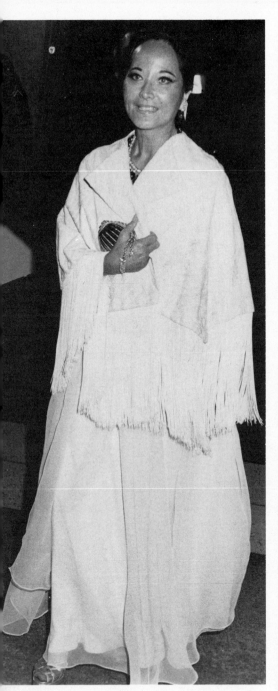

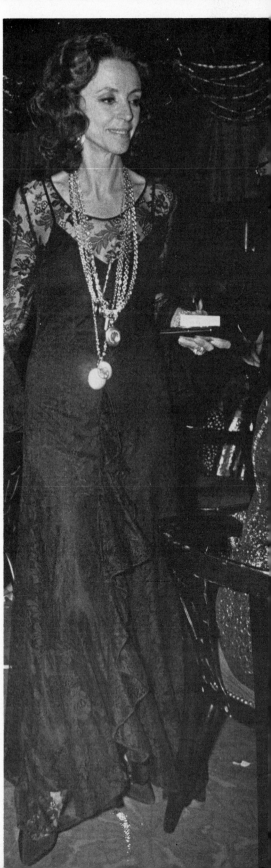

At the Academy Awards ceremonies, classic beauty Merle Oberon shows the effect of learning to take care of herself early in life. (*Women's Wear Daily*)

During a Rothschild party, Gloria Guinness table-hops as a way to avoid gastronomic temptations. (*Women's Wear Daily*)

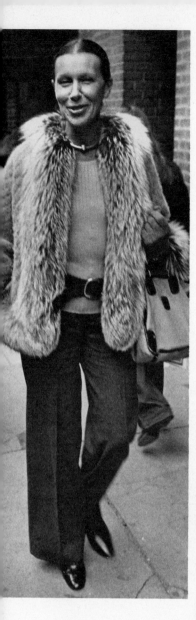

Looking great in her hip-huggers, Françoise de la Renta leaves a luncheon at Orsini's. (*Women's Wear Daily*)

Richard Burton, Elizabeth Taylor, and Princess Grace of Monaco at Liz's fortieth birthday party in Budapest. (*Women's Wear Daily*)

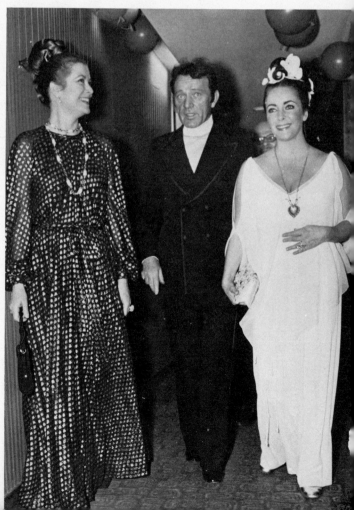

Perhaps it all depends on where you go. If you want to watch your weight, my advice is "go East." Were I ever to get fat, I would take the next plane to Ceylon. The food is uneatable. When I was there, I lived on papaya, king coconut, cashew nuts, and bananas and took long walks on the beach, and I've never felt so wonderfully skinny in my life.

Producer Franco Rossellini's theory is to go West and Middle East. "When I was in New York the last time, for fifteen days, I never had lunch out, only dinners," he says proudly. "At dinner, somehow, one manages to eat less. I lost six pounds and was so happy about it that when I came back to Rome I decided to eat only mozzarella cheese. I had mozzarella cheese until one day I almost fainted, so I started really eating again. Then luckily I had to go to Cairo and Luxor. In Luxor they give you the most dreadful rice, the most dreadful meat—the only choice is to diet. I lost another fourteen pounds."

For most of us, travel is the exception rather than the norm. We are not confronted all that often by a wide choice of unknown and possibly exotic restaurants. But if you work, you still eat out more often than not. In normal life, you are still invited out for dinner and you entertain. The prime consideration here is how often you do it. Once or twice a month? Every day? Four or five two-martini business lunches every week and you are in trouble. Three or more cocktail parties and private dinners per week, and again you are in trouble unless you learn to control yourself.

Given a choice, I think many professional women prefer to avoid mixing food and business during the day. While at *Vogue*, Diana Vreeland almost never went out for lunch and advises against it: "It only cuts your energy and vitality." French businesswoman Hélène Rochas adamantly concurs: "In the States, at least you don't have the French lunch. The men here still believe in it. They eat so much I wonder how they get through the day. When I was in business, I rarely made lunch engagements. I preferred to have appointments during working hours or over a relaxed drink in the evening."

I think she is right, for more reasons than one. Look at the expense-account bunch—they are, on the whole, a flushed and jowly lot. When a meal in a good restaurant is no longer a special treat but part of the daily routine, the only solution is quietly to cut back. You do not have to talk about it. You simply drink less, order the simplest thing you enjoy that's on the menu, and thereby feel better and keep your shape. It can be done.

Yves Vidal, who represented Knoll International in Europe, says he has not eaten alone for twenty years. His system: "No matter where you eat, and especially in restaurants, you don't have to take second helpings or eat bread or sweet desserts."

Earl Blackwell of Celebrity Service, whose job includes constant lunching with clients, uses similar restraint. "I have a very small breakfast. At lunch I order only one course and try not to drink anything more than a Dubonnet or a glass of wine. I enjoy dinner."

"I've had constant lunches and dinners for the past fifteen years," says Nicole Alphand. "My technique is to eat a little of everything, and I also have a diet day once a week or at least twice a month. The fact is I really like eating out. When I'm free to have a lunch all by myself, I don't go home. I go to Maxim's, where I have a table reserved. They know me and know I'll have only one course and coffee. They're quite happy with this and never look askance. One of my favorite lunches there is a hamburger with an egg on top. It's more restful to do this than to cross town to go home where I know my eye will spot too many things that have to be attended to and where, instead of relaxing, I'll wind up making lists between mouthfuls and giving orders."

The opposite of moderation is not only inflated lunches and overeating. It is also what is known as the grab-a-bite syndrome. Working under pressure, you get in the habit of settling for a sandwich, a Coke, coffee, or whatever else can be bolted down on the job. Celebrities, show-biz stars, government VIPs and their entourages, campaigning politicians, businessmen, journalists, doctors—you name it—all subject themselves to bouts of this.

"You always need a mental and physical cure after a film," says Elsa Martinelli. "You know, the lunch break can be at any hour—it depends on the weather and on how long it takes to shoot a scene. You arrive famished, more often than not with the summer sun beating down on your throbbing head, reach for your box lunch, tear it open, and what do you find? You find some dreadful piece of meat, hundred-year-old cheese, and reject fruit staring up at you. Marcello [Mastroianni] is convinced that no one eats worse lunches than actors on location."

I suspect that many people eat this terrible way out of habit rather than necessity. I also have the impression that many housewives, instead of fixing themselves something decent in between cleaning, committees, and kids, reach instead for the nearest convenience food, as if it took less time to open a can of worms than to prepare something fresh. You do not even have the excuse of external circumstances—you are not at the mercy of some fast-food service, you are in your own house! It is true that when I lunch at home I do not have to prepare it. Still I know that washing five leaves of lettuce and a sprig of parsley, scrubbing a carrot and slicing a tomato, and boiling two eggs or making an omelette do not exactly make you a slave in the kitchen. Furthermore, when cheese and apples exist, why choose soup and a sandwich?

Curiously enough, among the most entrenched victims of the grab-a-bite syndrome are the glamour-girl fashion models. Until they learn better, by collapsing on the job, they think that this aberrant pattern is as indispensable as their tote bag and book of photographs. London model-school director Cherry Marshall has come to the conclusion that if you have a good breakfast, skipping lunch is better than grabbing junk on the run. Models have to be thin, but they also have to have stamina, which does not come from sugar and starch. Eileen Ford, who valiantly lectures her girls on how to eat properly as well as moderately, always comes up with ketchup on her face.

"No matter what I say, in the beginning they all have the same habit. In between takes, they all insist on trying to make a cold, greasy cheeseburger and a milkshake do for lunch."

They will not do at all, and the habit brings on pounds and malnutrition. Fatty hamburger, plastic cheese, puffy bun, and sugary shake are a far cry from prime chopped beef with a fresh egg and a sip of wine for lunch at Maxim's. Most of us, to be frank, are not likely to lunch at Maxim's, but the principle of nutritious eating holds. When you work and lunch out five days a week, you cannot afford to eat non-food. If there is no pleasant place nearby to have a decent lunch, brown-bag it from home. A lot of secretaries do, and their bosses could learn a lesson from them. A hard-boiled egg, cottage cheese or yogurt, fruit, or half a broiled chicken or a few slices of ham from a takeout store are easily carried along. As for something to drink, what is wrong with water? If the municipal brew is polluted, try bottled water.

Then comes dinner. Theoretically you are supposed to eat less at night than at noon, but this almost never happens. In the States, where dinner is early, it does not really matter that it has become the principal meal. When it's cooked at home just for the family, you can still keep it nonfattening. The potential trouble lies in the custom of social gobbling in the evening. You come home, relax, have a drink, have friends over or are invited out—and eat like mad. Once a month? Fine. Several times a week? No good.

In Europe, particularly in France and Italy, social gobbling often takes place in a restaurant, where again it is up to you to choose wisely. Invited to a friend's for dinner, your only choice, if you care to exercise it, is restraint. At buffet dinners, which have become more common as servants and space dwindle, you can avoid the platters that spell extra pounds; nor is there any need to overload your plate as if you were never going to see food again. At sit-down dinners, which I must say are infinitely more pleasant, you hesitate to wave away a course and sit there with your empty plate staring up at you. Everyone is brainwashed to believe that saying no is a serious breach of good manners. In that case, mine are terrible. I know what things are bad for me, and when they are offered, I refuse.

Saying no, thank you, is the response, however. Never say you are on a diet. A pall of gloom will descend on the table as fellow guests realize that maybe they should be dieting too, and their only defense is to attack. Wanting to enjoy the abundance, they will all but force-feed you.

You can talk about any weird or painful disease at the dinner table—it is amazing how many people love to—but the sickness of overweight remains a taboo subject. In fact I sometimes think that one of the best secret-dieter's ploys is to pretend to be the victim of some dreadful malady that prevents eating, rather than confess to the admirable intention of trying to stay in shape. Having an amoeba, for example, is an excellent excuse. No one knows much about amoebas and how to feed their carriers. Moreover, if it seems in bad taste to bring disease to the table, you have a pure motive, and there are excellent precedents for doing so. To quote only one source, Vera Stravinsky has written of the custom:

> To the casual observer, Igor's behavior at table might seem somewhat odd, but the outstanding eccentricities, as doubtless they would be called, are almost common in Russians. Thus he appears to relish dinner-time discussions of liver, bladder and bowel troubles; but so did Tolstoy (see the Countess Sophia Tolstoy's *Journal*), and as the same unseemly inclination is manifest in so many Russians of my acquaintance, I wonder if it might not be

classified as a cultural trait. (One encounters it in the French, too, however, as in this description by the Goncourts of a dinner with Flaubert, Zola, Turgenev, Daudet: "We began with a long discussion on the special aptitudes of writers suffering from constipation and diarrhea.")

On the other hand, I have discovered that, without any effort, without the use of any distracting ploys such as the one I have ironically suggested, some people find dinner parties no poundage threat at all. On the contrary, for them dinner parties actually turn out to be diet evenings. It has to do with their mental attitude, which I wish I had and very much envy. (When I am with friends, I tend to bask in food as well as their presence.)

London's Georgiana Russell says, "I always eat less at parties. It's not out of nervousness, and I'm not a social butterfly. I'm too busy being talked to and talking."

Baroness Pauline de Rothschild, one of Europe's great hostesses, explains it beautifully: "Going out for lunch and dinner constantly is hopeless for your health, your body, and your mind. You get a feeling of food and overeasy life all around you that is disagreeable. A certain amount of sociability, however, will keep you thin in a curious way: listening, for instance. I cannot bring myself to listen to anyone at a dinner party with the lower part of my face filled out and the jaws chomping.

"While talking oneself, one can manage to speak with a small amount of food in one's mouth, as conversation would be immeasurably slowed down by swallowing first—remember Colette's instructions for the early table training of a successful young whore. Still, I'm sure that I leave many dinners having hardly eaten at all. If I eat a good deal in the beginning, I realize it is a commentary on the dinner's getting off to a slow start.

"At lunch, when I'm receiving, we have one course and maybe a sweet, and everyone is delighted. I take very little of it so I can have a second helping. If I didn't, everyone would say no. At night I have adopted the English habit of not having the first course passed around again. Then later, I like to stay on at the table because of the talk, and too much serving gets in the way."

It might be added that this emphasis on conversation and the human ingredients of a meal is based on the assumption that of course you are dining on good food. When London hostess Elaine Kennedy Gombault insists that what counts is to make people feel appreciated, you can bet that this is because she takes the planning of an interesting menu for granted. After that point what matters, indeed, is that Ingrid Bergman, sitting in a corner, be brought together with the shy man, off in another corner, who worked on *Anastasia*, or that Erté meet a great friend of Augustus John. However, all insistence that party success depends solely on the meeting of minds and the mix of people falls flat if the guests are not being fed well too.

Cappy Badrutt is the first to agree that going out three or four times a week is killing, especially in France, where the food is so rich.

"But let's not go to the other extreme, where you starve," she adds. "I went to a shoot where there were twenty-five people at dinner. We had four crayfish apiece, one glass of white wine, and one chocolate-covered prune. The hostess was very thin, and I could see why."

When entertaining, what can you do to maintain a comfortable balance? The first step is to cut down on the courses, and not just at lunch. Even at dinner the two-course meal has become standard. You need to have a good butcher and to select the freshest possible produce. Keep the main course simple, which is not the same as dull, and the dessert rich, or vice versa, though I do not know anyone who really likes a main course swimming in a sauce with herbs that scream for attention instead of being subtle.

What do well-known New York hostesses serve? Often a rack of lamb, a roast filet of beef, or a fine fish, salad, and for dessert a crème brûlée or a mousse, though more often it is a cheese tray and fruit in season, served raw, poached, or marinated in champagne. What else can you do, faced with the high price of meat? You skip meat. You can do a hundred things with poultry or eggs, and you can balance the starch of a huge rice or pasta dish with salad, cheese, and fruit.

Colette Lefort, French diet writer and journalist, is both flexible and strict about entertaining. For example, she thinks it better to serve fruit for dessert than something rich and sweet—whatever her guests' expectations—because they will feel better the next day. On the other hand, she suggests, when serving fish or asparagus, offering two accompanying sauces, one simple and one rich and giving your guests the choice. In the old French order, foie gras came after the first course(s) and meat. Now you can serve it first and eliminate a course. She also suggests starting with a soufflé, if your guests will be on time; otherwise a quiche, followed by lamb or chicken with a vegetable such as endive or peas, a salad, cheese, and fruit. (The enzymes in pineapple, by the way, help digestion.) You drink wine, but water is also on the table. The bread is country bread.

A stiff drink, a glass of wine, a beer, or a split of champagne before dinner—why not (unless you are still floating from lunch)? On the other hand, watching what you eat will not keep you thin if you drink yourself fat.

"After ten days in California, I looked at my husband and the rest of the group," says American-born Baroness Gaby van Zuylen. "The Americans, though attractive, looked appallingly fat—they all drink so much. You go to the golf club and it's 'Let's have a bloody Mary, or a Danish bull.' They make them so strong, they're impossible to finish: your tongue turns to cotton. This is followed by a sandwich that you couldn't possibly get through. You finish golf at four thirty and it is time for the next round. Even when you work, the hours are shorter in the States, and you start to drink so much earlier in the evening that everyone, especially the men, looks like a tub."

The baroness likes a drink; so does her husband; so do most people I know. We are not hard drinkers. If you care about your face, your figure, and your health, you cannot be. (I do not know how the myth got started that social drinking is fine, and the only time to worry is when you become a closet drinker. It is not who you are with or whether you're alone that matters; it is the quantity of alcohol consumed.) It does help not to nibble while drinking—avoid those cocktail tidbits like the plague, including the celery, which is invariably stuffed with something fattening. Cumulatively, the tidbits are as full of calories as the alcohol and ruin your appetite for serious food. Furthermore, if you do not nibble, you will want to have an honest meal sooner and will drink that much less.

"Sometimes I think they drink more in America than any-place in the world," says Ceezee Guest. "In Texas, they don't want the glass, they want the bottle. But even in places like Virginia, Philadelphia, and Boston, where I'm from, it's un-believable. Mind you, it may be changing now—the drunks die off early. The attractive people, the smart people, the ones who look well at forty-five, fifty, even sixty, drink little!

"When I have friends for dinner, I say that we eat at a quarter to nine and, with that in mind, come anytime you want. Inviting people early only means they get plastered. We have two rounds of drinks and that's it. We don't wait."

I am convinced that, when you're invited out, half of the fat and health battle is won if you do not stagger to the table. Good for Ceezee and good for every hostess who avoids seat-ing her friends at the table in a sodden lump.

Please bear in mind that it is mostly up to you to practice

restraint with food and drink, for the obvious reason that good hostesses, including myself, are not about to invite people over for an exercise in austerity. The hostess herself, if it is a small friendly dinner, may have her own diet dishes, which she does not inflict on anyone else. London-based Argentine beauty and hostess Maria-Marta de Santamarina has the discipline and social tact to carry this off beautifully. While you are busy with the bird and its accessories, she dips quietly into her brown rice. While you drink wine, she has a few sips of water. Needless to say, she also has the sense to order an abundant rice platter because everyone is curious and wants a taste. In your own house, I do not see why you cannot do what suits you as long as you do not make an issue of it. Madame de Santamarina, who is marvelously slender, has medical reasons for avoiding certain foods. Rather than stop entertaining, she limits herself but never her guests.

What she might serve but never eat at home, where alternatives are available, she succumbs to when invited out: "Pâté de foie gras is death, but, of course, I had some the other night."

If you truly must lose weight and can never deviate from broiled protein and raw greens, maybe it is easier not to face temptation. While under martial law, do not go out for dinner, which does not necessarily mean an early curfew. You simply regret to say that you have another engagement. You will try to break away early, and is it all right if you come after dinner? Usually it is.

When I entertain, it is not with restrictions in mind. I love to provide abundant fare, even if the family chokes for days on leftover food. I do not make special provision for friends who are on a diet or just not very hungry. I assume that, in that case, they will have the good sense to eat accordingly. The least I owe my guests is a feast for the eyes—and who knows? Maybe I have invited someone who is ready for a well-earned food orgy. How nice of him to want to splurge with me!

The cure for sporadic overindulgence is simple. The following day, or the first possible day within the same week, you compensate for the binge by eating very little and drinking even less, except for water. This is known as having your cake and keeping your figure too. Unless you act as if every night out were New Year's Eve, it works.

7

A Little Round Is Sound

I once asked George Plimpton what he thought about the beautiful people's classic dictum: "You can never be rich enough or thin enough." The writer and man-about-New York sniffed and all but snorted.

"There's only one answer to that," he replied. "Of course you can."

Needless to say, the money/body pronouncement, attributed to Gloria Guinness and Babe Paley among others, is more a *boutade* than an article of faith (though I confess that the first part of it appeals to me). As for thinness, again I am in favor, but not when it reaches manic proportions.

When I see someone who could be a real beauty if she lost a few pounds, I am not the false friend who says, "Darling, you look wonderful . . . it doesn't matter." I look at that moon face, note that thickening thigh, and itch to say get rid of them. On the other hand, I am over my adolescent longing for the down-to-the-bone model look. You can look fantastic in clothes, fantastic in a bathing suit when you have the freshness and supple skin of the early twenties, but there is a moment when the look turns dried-up and haggard. The thinness thing can go too far. It has gone too far when it has not only become unflattering but made you a nervous wreck. Everyone around you suffers from your weight obsession—suffers because you are always irritable or because your disapproval of more generous eating habits prevents everyone else in your immediate circle from enjoying food and drink that do not necessarily make *them* fat.

My plea is for equilibrium. While most fat people do not lose enough weight, there are those who, amazingly, get hooked on dieting and do not know when to stop. Everyone has heard horror stories of chic women who stick their fingers down their throat to reduce through vomiting, but anorexia, the refusal of food, is not confined to them. In extreme cases, you no longer have to resort to manual aid. You develop a conditioned reflex; what goes down must come up. It tears your insides out, of course. As for abuse of diuretics and pills and shots, why else do you think all those thin ladies used to be photographed in all the right places with the same identical smashing smile? They were smashed.

"A girl friend of mine who was overweight had absolutely genius pills," says Loulou de la Falaise. "Take half of one and you feel marvelous, but you don't sleep. You smile the whole time. It gets so you spend your entire life grinning and screaming if anyone says anything remotely funny."

Even without resorting to drugs, and possible breakdowns in consequence, a militant minority of women dedicate themselves to scrawniness through undereating. If they ever had an overweight problem, it was years ago. They now have a last-puritan compulsion to be gaunt, as if thinness were next to godliness.

"I had a woman in my office," says Dr. Fulvio Rossi, "who was down to ninety-four pounds and wanted to know how she could lose 5 more. She wasn't a midget, and when she wouldn't listen to reason, I threw her out. I wasn't about to help her lose weight when she needed to gain it."

Society columnist Suzy, whose business it is to observe the people she writes about, fell for the skinny cult herself but is now firmly against it. "When you're thin, you may look chic, but you don't look juicy—you don't look female," she says. "Certainly, after forty, 5 pounds over is better than 5 pounds under. I thought I was sensational at 103 until I saw my face in pictures. I'd had to lose weight, but I'd gone too far.

"I should have known better because I recognize the mistake in other women instantly. You know who I mean—she was terribly fat when young, so she went the other way, and now the bones in her back stick out, her hipbone is like a rock, and she has those little arms that look like strings. I saw her the other night, and she told me, 'I've never felt better in my life.'

" 'My God,' I thought, 'you've ruined yourself.'

" 'I'll never weigh more than 98 pounds again,' she said.

" 'What do you have for breakfast?' I asked. 'Orange juice and coffee?'

" 'Oh no, I have an egg,' she said.

"Can you imagine—she was talking about one egg, and she began to salivate. If you did this sort of thing and you came out beautiful, I could understand it. But if you come out bones?"

Suzy stopped herself in time. She prefers to watch her weight ("five pounds and I diet") than to beat the scales so thoroughly that she ends up the real loser. Overdieting is such a sterile pursuit. It may or may not be damaging to your health—some believe it lowers your resistance to stress and colds—but even if it is healthy, what is the point if you look a wreck? The only thin lady I know who does look divine is

Silvana Mangano, but with that bone structure you cannot go wrong.

"Silvana? Well, Silvana doesn't eat at all," says producer Franco Rossellini. "I don't know how she keeps alive. She swallows one salad leaf and takes a sip of *digestif* because she has eaten too much. I drink wine with meals. Don't you? Silvana has huge glasses of Fernet Branca with water. It's not only frightening, it's a problem. Before you take her out, you have to make sure they've got the stuff—a lot of restaurants don't."

People whose metabolisms make it a constant effort for them to keep their weight up to par will always tell you they feel better when they reach their ideal weight than when they are under the mark. Listen to them.

"The moment I'm unhappy, I lose weight—others swell like toads," says Gaby van Zuylen. "Even when I'm happy, I go thin. I think I was born this way. I was always the kind of child that mothers wanted to take home and feed. When I'm pregnant, I'm plump and nice; afterward I weigh even less than I did nine months before. I know that at 119 pounds I feel well, but I slip right back to 114.

"One winter I decided to do something about it. I was really thin and drawn—it must have been in January; that's the worry month when it seems that everyone dies. Gloria Guinness gave me the name of a doctor in Lausanne. I went up by train and took the taxi straight to his office. The doctor popped me on a couch, played with my tummy as if it were a piano, and said to give him three weeks and he'd fatten me up: 'We'll put tubes down and force-feed you.' I told him I'd like to think it over, walked straight to the station, and caught the next train back to Paris. No one's going to force-feed me."

"When people see how much I eat," says Elsa Martinelli, "sometimes they almost hate me. Poor darlings, it makes them suffer, and I can understand. If I had their problems, I'd weigh 200 pounds—I'd never learn self-control. As it is, I have to undergo treatment every year to keep my weight up. It's not a question of nerves—I have no trouble sleeping. I've tried going off cigarettes. That only made me neurotic, and I didn't gain any weight. My appetite is excellent.

"I've been going to Dr. Albert Creff now for seven years— he's the official dietician for French athletes. Every spring I take his shots, pills, and drops. The treatment helps you to assimilate your food. For my height, I should weigh about 128 pounds. Without Creff, I never get past 121, and I can assure you that 7 pounds mean a lot to your morale and well-being."

Betsy Theodoracopulos is another who drops weight very quickly unless she eats up: "Ten pounds can go in a flash, and the first place it shows is in the face." To be candid, neither the baroness, the actress, nor the New York socialite look skinny; each, in her own way, is an extremely glamorous, attractive woman. But that is the point. If they are aware that being too thin is no good, although it is their natural tendency, what is this ridiculous anti-flesh mania that makes some women diet to excess?

Scrawniness is not becoming, and certainly it is not sexy. Unless you have written off sex—which is your prerogative, if that is the way you feel about it—you might as well realize that men like something to grab. (Don't you?) They are not mad for fatties, but the ghoul look also puts them off. In fact, a recent research study carried out by William Shipman and Dr. Ronald Schwartz, two Chicago psychologists, involving thirty married couples, indicated that married fatties not only want to make love more often than their slender sisters, but, statistically, they do. The study pointed up a curious contrast between the supposed preference of men and the actual performance of women. The husbands were shown three female silhouettes: one ideally proportioned, the next plumper, the last plumper still. The men preferred the more slender silhouette. Yet when the wives were asked to state how often they had sex, the plump ones had the higher average and were

the only ones hoping to improve it. It is perhaps also signifi-
cant that the researchers did not even bother to include a
silhouette of an underweight woman, as if it were obvious that
no man would jump at that.

"Men hate the thin-lady type," says Georgiana Russell.
"They like a little meat. Did you see *Klute*? Do you remember
when Jane Fonda talks to the psychiatrist about caring for
someone for the first time in her life? She explains it with
gestures—gentle, open, rounded gestures—and the psychiatrist suggests that the word she is searching for is 'giving.'
There's also a sequence of shots taken of Jane Fonda from the
back. She's not bony at all, but she has a skinny back. My
immediate reaction was 'I'd love to be that thin.' The men
with me chorused, 'No, don't do it.' In a way, the lost round-
ness of youth is very sad."

Gil, the makeup wizard whose job is launching a thousand
faces, is adamant in his opinion. "Twiggy can be fun," he says,
"but I'd rather see Jane Russell. Women who diet are always
in such a bad mood. They're exhausted and, with their glassy
stares and the bags under their eyes, they might as well be on
marijuana. I can think of only one reason to stay on a stringent
diet—that's if you want a divorce and you can't get it. Try
chewing carrot sticks in bed."

"A girl's thinness is the last thing that attracts me to her,"
says Frederick (Frecky) Vreeland, suave, handsome first
secretary of the U.S. Embassy in Paris. "That wiry model look
automatically makes a girl unattractive to me, and any conversation concerned with weight is immediately repugnant.
There's no point in a woman's saying she's doing it for me—
I don't think girls should be overly thin. I'm all against it.

"Psychologically, it's terribly destructive to have this weight
thing gnawing away at you. I've known girls who had everything going for them, and they still couldn't stop being
bugged by it. Who gives a damn? It's a real hangup. I lived
four years in Morocco. In the Arab world, a woman is attrac-

tive for her flesh, not her bones. Flesh is sensuous, and how modern Western woman decided it's in to be thin is beyond me."

Before we all turn into Rubens models and whales, which is not what either he or I suggest, it might be added that the urbane Mr. Vreeland went through what he calls a fascinating experience: "A girl I spent two weeks with thought it would be a good idea to devote the time to going on a diet as well. So we combined getting to know each other with Dr. Stillman's Quick Weight Loss Diet. It was a gag. It was fun to do it *à deux* with a girl one cared for, even a sort of intellectual challenge to find ways to be on a diet and still eat to one's satisfaction.

"The diet is amazingly good. I lost a pound a day for ten days, to her immense displeasure. She used to watch me get on the scale and smile because I'd lost a pound—the punch line being that she gained weight."

Frecky adds that a week later he caught a disastrous cold and is sure it was because he had no resistance. He also adds (because, of course, he was asked) that he still sees the girl, who, as far as he knows, has stopped dieting. Personally, the idea of low-cal romance strikes me as a fantastic new angle on Eros. The particular diet they chose gives you a high-protein jolt, and who knows what a lift that could be?

"I went to northern Russia one summer to write about the Kiji wooden churches for *Vogue*," says Baroness Pauline de Rothschild. "I took an overnight train, and a very plump and beguiling peasant woman was curled up in the berth across from me. It set me to wondering whether we really cheat men from one whole element of a woman's body: the element of plenty. The line between string-bean charm and dried-up string is tenuous. Maybe there is a time in your life when you should be slightly heavier.

"In the back of our mind we have this image of those huge women in transparent gauzes who appear to resemble great sea elephants. We can't stand the idea anymore; it strikes us as a form of illness. Still, there are Venusian types who are meant to be slightly plump. Some old-fashioned women look so young—they've filled out the skin. If you are a woman who is looked at and renowned for her beauty, of course, you have to adhere to the perfect, slender criterion; you walk the chalk-line."

It is also a question of age. What you can get away with at twenty takes on a different character by the time you are forty. If you stay slim—which is not the same as thin—to be healthy, bravo! If you do it for aesthetics, again bravo! Who does not love to see a vigorous, flat-bellied, clear-eyed elder—a retired navy man, for example—out for a stroll, a spring in his step? Who does not love to see a trim, active older woman who holds herself more erect than we ever dreamed of and sits with a straighter back than we will ever have (as we slouch with relief on the nearest upholstered couch)?

Needless to say, one admires not just the proper weight but, above all, the carriage and superbly disciplined condition for the age. If you think that staying slim will, by itself, make you look young, forget it. You can fake it; with the right clothes and under the right lights you can avoid looking matronly or like a dowager, but when you hit the beach and the bedroom, age will out—and why shouldn't it? There is nothing criminal about turning forty, fifty, sixty, and more.

Italian beaches, for example, are rampant with aging play-boys trying to suck in the decline and fall of their skin and to mask their wrinkles with a tan. They are more or less the right weight, but a few extra pounds might give the tired dermis a buoyancy it sadly lacks. Were they heavier, of course, they might look more mature, which, come to think of it, is what they are supposed to be anyhow. I like a man to be in shape —and my husband is—but I do find it tiresome and silly for a man to pretend, just because he does not have a gut, that he is still one of the beach boys.

One popular theory holds that with each decade after twenty you should put on at least two pounds. This is summed up by the anonymous quote: "Baby, you can't win them all; after forty, it's your face or your ass and you've got to choose." The theory is also borne out by the common experience of watching a chic New Yorker or Parisienne from the back as she nips down the street or maneuvers through a cocktail party. She looks fantastic until, by chance, she turns around and that haggard face with the tension around the eyes comes at you like Methuselah in drag. Myrna Loy, for one, advises allowing yourself an extra five pounds so the face does not look so ravaged. She is not the only glamorous woman who thinks that way.

"I believe you have to mellow," says Arlene Dahl. "Dolores del Rio thinks a few pounds are essential. Otherwise, the neck gets scrawny, and the bloom goes off the face. You can always camouflage your figure, but you can't hide your face. Even a face-lift never gives back the bloom."

The word of caution here is that putting on weight is only too easy as you grow older, and losing it grows correspondingly harder. Beware of menopause fat. Once on, you may get stuck with it. Filling out for bloom may have its charm; full-blown middle-aged spread is less appealing and usually unhealthy. It is up to you to determine the point of no return, just how far to go and why. Maybe your reasons for letting go within limits at any age have nothing to do with beauty. I may disagree, but as long as you know what you are about, your point of view is valid.

"Everything in the world I love to do—writing, painting, giving food, and talking—is done seated," says Fleur Cowles. "I would be tremendously thrilled to be ten pounds less if it were handed to me as a gift. No one will hand it to me, and I'm not about to change my life to achieve it. Ten pounds less is part of the beauty package I'm not in; it would take a sort of total vanity that I just haven't got. Ultimately, people are weighed and measured by their reputations. If you are known as a beautiful woman, you have to stay beautiful. Hardworking professionals, on the other hand, do not have to conserve something that at best is ephemeral. It's one of their luxuries.

"I don't drink, I don't smoke, I don't use bread in the house. If I'm not lunching with people, I might just have an egg. Breakfast is a cup of tea, except on Sunday morning at our country house in Sussex. There we spend two or three hours around the table in our robes. We have the papers; we debate and we discuss. So many things come out over pâté and griddle cakes—it's the most delightful communal gathering I know, and if, in the end, one eats a little more, so what?

"My weight has been the same for the past ten years, and until it becomes a medical issue I'm going to ignore it. I am well aware that people who are obese have terrible problems, but obesity is not the case at hand. What we are discussing are the 'ten vain pounds' you can do without or live with just as well. I have mine for convivial reasons."

After her first bout with a fat farm, Liz Carpenter, former right arm of Lady Bird Johnson, concluded that some people are born to look like Queen Victoria and she is one of them. In an article for *McCall's*, she figured that she has about thirty pounds to spare. On the other hand, she has been married for twenty-seven years and asks herself, "Doesn't love mean never having to say you'll diet?"

Coco Chanel, whose pearls of wisdom multiply now that she is dead, just as her suits were copied while she lived, is supposed to have had little patience with a client who wailed that she couldn't lose weight. Once she had ascertained that the client was happily married, Chanel told her to let well enough alone.

Actually, the decision does not depend on having or not having a man. It depends on being aware of your physical type and your priorities. I am all for staying in shape. Personally, I have no tolerance even for "ten vain pounds" if they are on me. Most of my friends feel the same way. We are conditioned to eating for slenderness and could not stand ourselves any other way.

But what if beauty is not your forte? If your basic structure —the one you already had by your late teens—is bosomy, hippy, and curvy, with short legs and arms, should you struggle against genetic odds to become a sylph? I doubt it. In other words, not only do I find the compulsive dieting of the "thin-lady syndrome" a caricature of the slender ideal, I also question, when the cards are stacked against you, the advisability of striving toward that ideal. I do not say go ahead and eat your boxes of chocolate, be obese, who cares! We all know that obesity is an invitation to high blood pressure, diabetes, and heart disease and usually means ugly!

I refer, on the contrary, to minor overweight. As long as your keep it minor, it may be better, in some cases, to live with it, placing the emphasis more on exercise and muscle tone than on a vain attempt to diet to the perfect proportions you will never have. This is known as making the best of your type instead of being the last long-distance runner in a race you cannot win. It assumes, of course, that you are eating sensibly and not transforming the discovery that you are an endomorph into an excuse for becoming a slob. You are fighting the good fight, staying at the optimum weight for your shape. If you are a few pounds, repeat, a few pounds over, dress for them and enjoy them. To quote a *Vogue* mind opener: "I'll grow my mind. I'll grow my energy. I'll grow my stamina. My weight can stay where it is."

8

Baby Fat Has to Go

You are an adult. You may be thin, fat, just right—or somewhere in between. Because you are an adult, your weight, no matter what you say, is strictly up to you. No one makes you eat. But what about your children, who depend on you for meals? If they are tubs, are you pretending it is only baby fat? What about your teen-agers, grown unwieldy or wan on food jags? Can you intervene?

Quite possibly you have always justified your own overweight with the old wives' tale that fat runs in the family. It turns out, in the light of recent research, that you are right. It also turns out—and there goes your excuse—that fat in the family does not mean fat is inevitable. What Mom—to say nothing of Dad and the experts—never prevented for you, a battle with the scales, you can prevent in part for your children.

Sorry, but it does appear that the biggest help is to set the example yourself. According to a study cited by Norman Joliffe, M.D. (in *The Prudent Diet*), when both parents are fat, 70 percent of their offspring are likely to have an eventual weight problem as opposed to only 10 percent when both parents are lean. Other statistics indicate that from 69 to 80 percent of overweight cases reveal a family history of obesity.

Therefore, when you and your gross ancestors seem to have produced a pear-shaped child, your first reaction is to say that very little can be done. Allah has spoken. It is written in the genes. I have no doubt that eventually some biologist will come up with serious evidence that blood will tell and that heredity does indeed play a part in a tendency toward over-weight. Certainly we seem to pass on basic body structure, whether you call it ectomorph, mesomorph, and endomorph for slender, medium, and large frames, or are content instead with simply identifying the family barrel chest as it rolls down through the generations.

"Don't you think you're born with a certain chemistry in your body?" asks a New York socialite. "I have two children; one is hard and scrawny, craves fruit, doesn't like sweets, and is very athletic. The other will always be heavy. My doctor has said so. He can tell by feeling the flesh. The little one has a sweet tooth. He's also got those enormous Mediterranean hips, just like his father. Do you know that my husband even had stretch marks in his teens?"

Most mothers notice such differences in their children. I notice it in my own teen-agers: my son has no problem, but my daughter has always had to watch her weight. Still, there is no conclusive proof that you are born to fat and will always have to fight it. It has been demonstrated, for example, that yellow-haired mice inherit an elevated appestat, but we are not yellow-haired mice! In the nature versus nurture contro-versy, we have to concentrate on nurture. That we can con-trol.

Fat starts in the cradle if the hand that rocks it also gives the infant too much food. One of the few points of agreement between pediatricians and diet experts is that the big, bouncing baby is not necessarily healthier than his smaller peers. Mothers know this by now, yet still continue to dote on beautiful fat babies with dimpled hands, triple chins, and legs like the Michelin tire man's. For fear of neglecting anything that helps the baby grow, they overdo.

Recent investigation by Dr. Jules Hirsch and several Rockefeller University colleagues has revealed that obese adults have not only bigger fat cells than people of average weight, but more of them. How did this come about? Everyone is born with much the same percentage of fat cells.

The Hirsch theory, based in part on an experiment with infant rats, some fed lavishly and others fed less well, is that early gorging creates the excess number of cells. These, in turn, "cry out" for excess food and once you have got them, you are stuck with them. (From what I understand, fat cells do not have nerve endings that scream out to be fed, and appetite is mostly in the mind. Still, you never know, and the fat cell theory is one more reason not to overpower a tiny child with food.)

Undernourishment, which, if protracted, can lead to brain damage, is a serious problem in Third World countries where from 60 to 70 percent of the children suffer mild to chronic malnutrition. As Dr. Neil Solomon, among other nutrition experts, has pointed out, the children of the poor in affluent societies can also be affected by protein deficiency because of the relatively high cost of protein foods such as meat, poultry, and fish. At the same time, a recent study by University of Pennsylvania researchers would indicate that children in poor white families are likely to be fatter than rich youths, although there is a "surprising incidence of overweightness in young children in general." In other words, in the overall picture, our children may be getting the wrong food and too much of it, but they are not underfed.

If your growing baby is normally round and lunges for his

Pablum, there is no need to fret. If he does not have an eating or digestion problem and is not roly-poly, you must be doing something right. But if he is a burly bruiser, check with your pediatrician, who might advise a cut in the starch and sugar department.

In one sense, I am all for prepared baby foods, with the exception of fruit (because it really takes no time to grate an apple). They may be slightly less nutritious and contain possibly dangerous additives, but if they are rejected you cannot feel resentful about all the effort you have put into preparing the baby's meal from scratch. On the other hand, when you have been chopping and sieving and straining away, to see the result spit out can make you very annoyed. Try jars. A few preservatives are better than a nervous uproar.

Above all, when an infant is not hungry, and you know it is not because he has had too many sweets, leave him alone. He is not going to waste away before the next meal. So you throw out a bit of meat, five spoonfuls of spinach, and a dab of grated fruit (it is not always worthwhile or safe to keep them) because the price of force-feeding is steeper. Nothing could be more grotesque than the game of the zooming spoon, still prevalent in Italy. This consists of jollying "il bimbo" into finishing his meal by holding a filled spoon aloft and making it fly in circles until it lands in the unsuspecting mouth. When the child is old enough to get off his chair and run, this game can progress all over the house.

Down with the clean-plate fallacy! It should have gone to the grave with Grandma. I was raised on it and therefore made quite sure that my children were not. It was one of the iron laws of the German nannies. The one who took care of me insisted upon it. (A word to the wise in passing: if you rely on nannies or *au pair* girls, make sure their ideas on feeding agree with yours. If the clean-plate fallacy rules at nursery school or the day-care center, the effect is less dramatic because only one meal a day is involved.) As a small child I was astounded, when visiting with friends, to discover that their English nannies taught instead that you must always leave a little something "for Mr. Manners." It was not polite to clean your plate. That sounded like freedom at last! Mind you, I do not really find it necessary for a child to leave food on the plate. There are other ways of attesting to civilized manners. I simply feel that as far as old-fashioned, rigid systems go, it is more sensible to place the emphasis on not being a pig than to risk making a child one by insisting that he eat all available food.

We all know that toddlers and growing children should have three regular meals a day. We also know that the meals should feature varying combinations of dairy products (including cheese), meat, eggs, whole-grained cereals, green and yellow vegetables, and fruit—the vegetables and fruit, to my mind, should be bought fresh and served raw, if possible. In Latin countries there is less emphasis on milk past infancy, with reliance placed instead on other dairy products—yogurt and "white" cheeses such as petit Suisse, ricotta, and mozzarella—for protein and calcium. Balancing the diet by the end of the day, or even in the longer run, is the most realistic aim. Children can have their anti-meat days without withering away. It is up to you to find an acceptable protein substitute —in pill form if need be—if the anti-meat days stretch into months.

"My children were raised in California in an era of greater permissiveness," says sculptor Marcia Panama, who now works in London. "For a year—it wasn't that long, but it seemed a year—my daughter would eat only bacon, ripe olives, and raw spaghetti, and drink only milk. Isn't that strange? She was about two years old when it happened.

"I think that, rather than put up a battle over food, you have to remember that nothing lasts forever. Slowly, you impose by example. You not only give them healthy food, you eat it too. I'm half rabbit, for instance. I always have salad and I swear by watercress. I like meat and I'm not big on sweet things. My daughter as well as my son fell into this pattern when they were still young. Of course, when they went away to school they binged on terrible stuff, but I see they've come back to normal now that they are old and decrepit [translation: in their twenties]."

I am sure that if my own daughter had pulled a food strike at age two, I would have had a fit. Viewed objectively, however, I feel Marcia is right. Although the ideal is a balanced diet, forgo it if it means making food an emotional issue. Better raw spaghetti than spinach if the spinach has to be force-fed. (We have all heard beautiful stories like the one about the little girl who hid her spinach, then strained it through the screen door when no one was looking or—my favorite one of all—the enchanting little bitch who dumped hers in the piano.)

Although some children never have eating problems, most do from time to time—problems, that is, from your point of view, because you fear they are not eating enough, are eating too much, or are choosing the wrong foods. Even if you are right, they come around much quicker if the atmosphere is not emotionally charged. Start sabotaging their appestat by making them eat when they are not hungry, and you cause more grievous trouble. No food is good for you if you do not feel like eating it.

Preparing three meals a day is a job, and a little professional detachment goes a long way. If you do not work outside the house, you probably did at one time and might remember that no matter how good you are at a job, there are times when your efforts are not in the least appreciated. As a housewife who cooks, you do not have the compensation of a weekly check and therefore may be tempted to expect payment for your work in emotional coin: If you love me, eat what I have made for you. In recent American fiction, the "Yiddisha Momma" has come to personify this smothering, stuffing approach, but in all probability it is mainstream rather than an ethnic characteristic.

To test his growing independence, a child is going to rebel against some aspect of his daily routine, and he will hit where it seems to hurt most. If you really care about his health and future looks, do not let the table become the battleground. Transfer the ego clash to another arena, like keeping his room neat or his shoelaces tied, but keep the pressure off eating.

Above all, never use food as a weapon or a reward. We all rely to a certain extent on "the shut-up biscuit" to obtain some peace and quiet, especially when traveling with young children. But it soon becomes a habit and you shove a cookie in a mouth at the first annoying interruption; the kid gets hooked on sweets, and the weapon turns against you. You have prepared the taste buds for the subsequent on-slaught of TV advertising, with its emphasis on packages and bottles of sugar and starch, additives, and other rich rewards. You have also set up the perfect conditions for blackmail. Every time you take the child out with you, the gimme-gimme wail goes up; you hate to look like a harsh mother in public and find yourself buying some piece of gar-bage for immediate consumption. You wind up coming home from the supermarket with a ton of non-foods that the child, not you, has chosen. (So I am told—happily, I never went through that ordeal.) No wonder women are beginning to petition supermarkets for supervised play areas where they could drop their children. No wonder most markets turn a deaf ear.

Who needs ten varieties of cereal (to be eaten with sugar)? Yet how many mothers wind up with at least that many on the kitchen shelf? Actually, it was the day that a New York friend of mine realized that nine different breakfast food boxes had insidiously crept into her cupboard that she rebelled.

"This is nonsense," she said. "Let the little monsters feel deprived because they are not munching the same glop as the kid on the screen or their friends down the street. Who is in control here, anyway?"

I know it is far more difficult to resist commercial pressure in the States than it is in Europe, where television is not yet the great baby-sitter and prepared foods are still in the minority. Our television day is shorter, with fewer channels; the commercials are grouped and on the whole are adult-oriented. A generation of young Italians, for example, is growing up with *Carosello,* a concentrated ten-minute advertising orgy. Its closing theme song, which signals bedtime for the grammar school contingent, is amusingly done but deals more in detergents, soaps, and apéritifs than in messages beamed directly at children. We are spared early conditioning to processed fatteners.

Who's in charge here? No amount of industrial and social pressure is going to make you buy food you do not approve of. If the kids do not know any better, you certainly should, and placing all the blame on advertising is a cop-out. Children fall easy prey to advertising only if you have already conditioned them by using food as a weapon, or even worse, as a reward.

"If you're a good girl, I'll get you an ice cream. . . ."

"Eat up, or you won't have any dessert. . . ."

"There's something in Daddy's pocket for you. . . ." (And rest assured it is candy, not an apple.)

Why is it that when you prepare an excellent, simple dinner, this is taken as a matter of course? But when you bake a cake or make a pie, you are queen for the day. Is it really the children's fault, or is it yours and your husband's? Are you passing on your own childhood conditioning?

Grace Mirabella, editor of *Vogue,* says, "To this day, when I have worked very hard and feel tired, I am terribly prone to eat sweets. I still feel I deserve them; they were the prize you earned as a child for being good. It's such a bad habit, and once instilled, it's very hard to break."

We know, or think we know, that sugar and sweets are no good for children—or for anyone. The sweet tooth, only too often, is a tooth with a cavity. Full of sweet snacks, a child neglects the meat and greens and fruit he needs, or if he laps up the good and the bad together, he gets, not stronger, but fatter.

Much as I believe in sustaining and rewarding children, I fail to see why it has to be done with sugar and starch, nor am I convinced that there is any compulsive physiological reason for a child to prefer them. It may be a coincidence, but most of the women I know who have never had a weight problem —give or take five pounds—recall distinctly that they never liked sweets, even as children. They remember, perhaps because it soon became part of family legend, that they were the ones who filched the dill pickles instead.

One method of putting junk food in its place is to ration the sweet stuff, a method often employed by parents when their children reach nursery or grammar school age. At that point, no matter how careful one has been at home, overexposure starts, and you cannot hope to fight all the candy bars and other kids in the world. I am not against the rationing system, as long as it does not work against itself by heightening the appeal of the almost "forbidden fruit." An acquaintance of mine, who is a compulsive chocolate eater and has a weight problem, still recalls how she would wait all day for the two chocolate kisses her father would give her when he came home. (One wonders whether she got them if she had been naughty.) In other words, if you are going to ration, do not make a big issue of it, and let the child eat his allotment for the day whenever he wants to.

The system works better when the youngster knows how to count and handle small change. In that case, he is given a specific small sum every day (a week is too long) as his gum–soft drink–popcorn–ice cream–candy allowance. It should be made quite clear that the sum does not cover all of these and that it is up to him to choose. He can blow it on one item, stretch it out, or hoard it up. The emphasis goes off the junk food itself; rationing becomes a game, and it is amazing how fast a child learns to comparison shop in the neighborhood and assert his consumer interest, a skill we might all acquire. It also helps, when feasible, for the parents of close playmates to agree on the sum to be spent.

Needless to say, the child's allowance should not be padded out by access to goodies at home. You should not keep cookies, soft drinks, and candy within reach; in fact, most of the time you should not have them in the house. Surely you do not eat and drink them often, do you? If so, how is your weight these days and how are you setting that golden example?

Bowls of fruit, seeds, and nuts can be left up for grabs instead. Children love snitching from a fruit bowl—it is not as if you were asking them to make do with something dreary. (There is one thorn in this rosy solution, and I am afraid that you are stuck with it; no matter what quick disposal schemes you impose, bits of shell, rinds, pits, and cores still turn up in the oddest places all over the house.)

Should all such reasonable approaches fail, one drastic remedy remains. It is not recommended for toddlers; in fact, it is dangerous for a tiny child. Your sturdy, ornery eight- to twelve-year-old will survive and get in one dramatic moment the point that has escaped him after years of your patient effort. I refer to the blitzkrieg. When a child's craving and whining for a particular food becomes insupportable, let him have whatever he wants in bulk. You point out, as you have always said, that too much makes you sick, but let him determine his own "too much"; when the almost inevitable happens, however, please forget the I-told-you-so's. No smirks allowed, and do not rub it in.

"My mother didn't fool around," a prominent New York lawyer still remembers. "Rather than prolong the agony of hold out one day, give in the next, she got my brother and me each a gallon of ice cream and sat us down in front of them. 'Okay,' she said, 'you win, and I dare you to finish it.' We turned green.

"Another time, she did the same thing with watermelon. I guess we must have been determined little bastards. One lesson wasn't enough. My mother got the ripest, biggest Jersey melon she could find, and in those days they were as sweet as they were big. We almost polished it off. After eighteen trips to the bathroom, we got the point. Do you know, I'm not a big eater to this day."

The emphasis so far has been on preventive measures: how to keep children from acquiring bad eating habits and an overly emotional attachment to food. Save the child from baby fat and chances are you save the future adult from obesity. I have concentrated on snacks and sweets because that is where trouble often begins. As for meal plans, once children are past the early years and if their weight is normal, they should eat basically the way you do.

Actress Arlene Dahl, for example, says she tries to make sure her children have protein, one yellow and one green vegetable, and fruit at every meal. They also take a vitamin supplement. A favorite lunch is a cheese soufflé and a mixed green salad, and a favorite dessert is sliced fresh fruit with a sprinkling of grated coconut.

"In California we have fig, avocado, and orange trees, which is great for the children," she says. "Everyone in the house likes to cook—my husband and son prepare surprise dinners together—and because we like to eat, we definitely frown on TV dinners. Our idea of a Saturday supper is Norwegian meatballs (with wheat germ replacing the bread crumbs). My husband and I don't drink hard liquor. We drink wine, and the children are allowed a glass. Even Sonny (the baby) takes his vitamins with a sip of Bordeaux. We rarely have sweets, but my daughter stops off on her way home from school for a candy bar."

London socialite the Hon. Mrs. Vere (Pat) Harmsworth

says that she gives her children black molasses, yeast, and multi-vitamins because she believes in them and takes them herself.

"Mostly I try to have them start and end each meal with something fresh," she says. "I never let them eat white sugar or white bread, and I try to get as much petit Suisse into them as I can. But when the nannies give them jam sandwiches, I close an eye. You have to have some indulgence."

Baroness Gaby van Zuylen says she has only a few rules, but she does try to stick with them. "I do the menus with the chef for the children as well as for us," she explains. "Obviously, they don't have a lot of fried foods. No one should. I don't let them eat between meals. They are given as much orange juice as they want, but they're not allowed Cokes until they're twelve—don't ask me why—and then only one a day. I do make the children eat a solid breakfast, which includes porridge in the winter. I'm absolutely adamant on this."

But what if your growing children have turned out to be little fatsos? What if you take a hard look one day and suddenly realize that what should be a firm little body is soft and puffy instead? You do not know where you have gone wrong, but obviously you have. The first step is to acknowledge it and not just pretend that the youngster's overweight is either normal or will melt away by itself.

If the overweight is moderate, the question to ask is whether the child gets enough exercise. A generation or two ago the question never had to be asked in suburb, small town, or country. In the city it was already pertinent, if less imperative: there was always stickball and running away from the cops who broke up games that got in the way of traffic. There also were gang wars, but the latter, which still exist, are not what I had in mind.

If children no longer walk to school or anywhere else (because they jump in the car with you), if they cannot run wild in relatively safe conditions, if the fields are built up, the streams polluted, and the streets a menace, it is not their fault. It is yours and your parents'. More and more, young children are reduced to organized sports and games in organized places, which cost money and necessitate the bore of either hauling them back and forth or arranging for other people to haul them. In continental Europe, where there are almost no playground or extracurricular sports in the public school system, the situation is even worse.

Thin kids and fat ones alike need exercise, and lack of it can be the start of a vicious circle. Even a well-balanced, non-excessive diet may lead a youngster into fat if his energy output is insufficient. Once a child is overweight and taunted by his playmates for awkwardness and slow reflexes, he moves even less. Bombarded by food ads as he sprawls in the comforting dark in front of the TV, he compounds the problem by munching as he passively watches his heroes' adventures in between the commercials. (Do you and your husband munch and swill in front of TV at night?)

It is well known that the overprotective mother who force-feeds her child is also the mother who fears for his life the moment he climbs on a bike or stands up on a swing. Most probably this is not your case. You simply have no place where the child can play off his energy—every day is like a cooped-up rainy day at home. I have no miracle solution. Circumstances vary far too much to establish feasible guidelines. I only repeat that you cannot build a firm young body unless you make sure that somehow your child has exercise as well as reasonable eating habits.

Mild overweight in children can also be due to the necessary filling-out periods that precede growth spurts. A slight weight gain between ages seven and nine is common, though it may be due to a more sedentary life—sitting at school, the discovery of the pleasure of reading, math, or chess, scrapbooks and collecting. Another common fluctuation occurs in prepuberty, especially among girls starting to develop breasts and menstruate. In general, the youngster grows into his weight.

But never assume. As soon as you see him fat, take the child to the pediatrician for advice. Let him decide whether you should ignore the extra weight or help the child get rid of it either right away or gradually. Whatever diet or method your pediatrician proposes will not work unless you too cooperate. In other words, those few potato chips, that small extra helping "that won't hurt" do make a difference. In the rare instances where an endocrine disorder is the culprit, taking the child to a pediatrician is the only right step.

"Endocrine dysfunctions can be corrected medically and with growth," says Dr. Fulvio Rossi. "The important thing is to catch them in time—between ages eight and ten. They are rare. I see lots of fat children, and in my experience the problem is usually emotional rather than glandular."

Bad eating habits, use of food as blackmail, lack of exercise, defective glands—you name it. No matter what the cause, nip it in the bud. Do not raise your children to be fat, and remember that the infancy through pre-teen years are crucial. It is much easier to brainwash your children to eat both little and right when they are under your wing than it is to correct them later on. A taste for raw vegetables and fruit, broiled meat, eggs, and cheese, when acquired early, lasts through life. Even Dr. Frederick J. Stare of Harvard, who defends the processed American way of eating more heartily than most experts I know, admits that thousands of young people would do better in school if they ate the right food. (One of his pet pleas is for adequate breakfasts.)

Once the foundation is laid, however, do not expect eating problems to simply vanish. Be prepared, on the contrary, for rather startling aberrations, especially in your children's late adolescence. This is the time for food jags, fad eating, anxiety stuffing, and even starving in order to look like a model. It is the time, above all, for questioning everything, if not for outright rebellion against family and other Establishment strictures. You delude yourself if you think that while they are protesting your spiritual and political values, your teen-agers are going to keep up their strength by eating properly. Maybe they think that you don't look so hot, so what is the use?

So far I have been lucky. I have not had too much trouble, and I have five teen-agers in the house with my own and my stepchildren. Four of them are girls, which may make it easier, because of girls' concern with being attractive. When my own daughter, who puts on weight easily, turned twelve, I took her aside for a little talk.

"It is clear," I said, "that you'll grow, but you are not going to be very tall. You can be a pocket Venus, but that means you cannot afford to put on weight—there's no place for it to go except wrong. I have raised you to know how to eat, so if you get fat, it's your own fault, and I won't want to look at you."

I know this sounds terribly harsh, and I'm really not such a dragon. Nevertheless, I think that with a girl that age, pussyfooting gets you nowhere, especially since, in this case, my daughter was going off to boarding school, where she would have to set her own limits. Better to be completely honest than to have her suffer through a painful, dumpy adolescence.

We discussed the foods you need and those you do not. Since then my daughter has had an occasional bout with extra pounds, but nothing that could not be coped with easily during vacations at home. I have never allowed her either to try drastic diets or to use any sort of diet or thyroid pill. In highly controlled situations they may be feasible, but you do not leave them to the discretion of a teen-ager (or of most adults). The temptation to abuse them is too great.

One of my stepdaughters was definitely overweight when she first came to live with me. During school vacation, with the stress of grades off her back, I set up a regimen for her:

Breakfast   Tea with lemon and honey

Lunch   About 3 1/2 ounces of spaghetti, weighed un-
               cooked (sauce to vary from day to day)
               2 veal cutlets or other lean meat (more if
               wanted)
               salad vinaigrette
               1 peach

Dinner   5 ounces of hard cheese of her choice
               OR 5 ounces of fat-trimmed ham and cheese
               OR 2 boiled eggs and cheese
               salad vinaigrette
               fruit

I did not calculate calories: I was not trying to see if she could add. I wanted her to get in the habit of eating the right sort of food, simple but deliciously prepared. For example, I think it is better to have a good salad—either lettuce alone or mixed—dressed with olive oil, salt, pepper, and vinegar or lemon than to cut out the olive oil and make the salad less enjoyable. In the long run, the idea is to get hooked on salads. No bread was allowed because spaghetti was included. Snacks, sweets, and soft drinks were taboo. There was no limit on the amount of water; in fact, she was encouraged to drink it when thirsty.

My stepdaughter was thirteen at the time. She lost twenty pounds in two months. Her meals required no special preparation. She could eat with the other children, whose meals, though less restricted in quantity, were basically the same. She did have to lose overnight her American habit of constant raids on the kitchen. It was less difficult for her living in an Italian household, where regular meals are important but no one hugs the refrigerator.

Needless to say, I spelled out what is fattening, what is not —a few starchy foods are needed for balance, but schedule them carefully and keep sweets to a minimum, preferably in the form of honey and fruit, providing natural sugars.

After two months, when she went off her diet, I saw her reaching for a second bun at breakfast.

"Oh, is it fattening?" she asked, aware she had been caught in the act.

"Listen," I said, "by now you know how the game is played. Let's not start the diet thing again. You can eat a little of everything now. Where buns are concerned, little is very little, and don't you forget it."

Knowing teen-age contradictions, it should come as no surprise that it is precisely this stepdaughter, the least disciplined of the three, who has vague ambitions to become a model. She will be tall enough, and her face could be photogenic, but she does not have the body structure for modeling. I am not trying to slim her down for what in her case, as I have explained to her, photographs in hand, would be an illusion of a career. My intention is to help her become the healthy, tall, and well-shaped young woman that she will revel in being.

I had her lose weight gradually—about two-and-a-half pounds a week over two months—for several reasons. The first is that active teen-agers need energy, and I did not want her to cut down on sports while reducing. The main reason, however, was to get her onto a sensible eating pattern she could enjoy. My objection to crash diets, for teen-agers, as well as adults, is that they are palliatives, not basic reform.

Nagging a teen-ager about food—too much, too little, or too far-out—is a waste of breath unless you have something better to offer, from his point of view as well as yours. Isolating him by inflicting a diet, even one prescribed by a doctor, so different from regular family fare that it seems a cruel and unfair punishment only invites cheating.

With girls, food problems are said to reflect conflicts about the best way to be a woman: what is truly attractive; what really matters? Elaine Kennedy Gombault advises flexibility.

"There was a period when I kept putting my daughter on diets. We tried everything. Then she fell in love and anxiously asked her boyfriend whether he thought she was a little overweight. He told her, 'No, I think you're perfect.' So she immediately lost ten pounds."

Jo Scott, a psychologist at the Metropole Hydro in Brighton, describes a classic case of the young girl grown obese to spite Mom as well as herself. In the favorable conditions of the farm, the patient lost weight, but every time her hyperactive, hyperthin mother came to visit, the girl's first reflex was to sneak out and load up on chocolates.

At least the mother had the sense to appeal to a third party, in this case a clinic. When your criticism, no matter how justified, of a teen-ager's looks or weight is resented and rebuffed, outside influences may still carry the day. Certainly you need outside help if your daughter goes to the opposite extreme and refuses food. Teen-age anorexia nervosa, though rare, may start with a crash effort to slim that gets out of hand until non-eating is compulsive. Some girls have literally starved themselves to death. I would always watch a dieting daughter, particularly one who diets on her own initiative, to see that she knows when to stop. (Boys rarely reach anorexia nervosa.) I am no advocate of the big bottom and expansive thigh, but you have to take body build and sex into account. Females have more cushion below the belt, and that is always the last fat to go. Better to take a size larger in blue jeans than starve yourself.

Since I have never had to face it, I have no idea what I would do if a sixteen-year-old of mine suddenly embraced the most drastic form of macrobiotics or turned strict vegetarian overnight. I suppose, as with pot, it would depend on how far he went and how he looked and functioned. A teen-ager is not a baby. He spends far less time at home, and you cannot be bodyguard anymore. Most food fads, given a trial, are soon abandoned out of boredom. Should one prove tenacious and visibly harmful, then intervene and insist on a checkup. The results determine what to do next, and you have avoided fruitless opinionated arguments.

Incidentally, improper food is to blame for malnutrition and weight problems, but not for acne. Diet alone will not clear up the skin. If you ban greasy foods and sweets, it will help a teen-ager with his shape, but it may do nothing to alleviate that other bane of adolescent appearance—all those ugly pimples. For them you need a doctor more than diet.

"To tell the truth," says Dr. Michael Kalman, a skin specialist, "there has never been any proof that any food has caused anyone to break out. The oil glands in the skin are the fundamental cause. Some people's are overactive because of heredity or hormonal balance. There are certain foods that people commonly associate with acne: chocolate, sharp cheeses, nuts, anything with iron in it, such as types of seafood, shellfish, spinach, and melons. Abolish them, get fresh air and exercise, but I repeat, there has never been a good study to prove that it makes any difference. You can treat acne with medications, including Vitamin A acid for severe cases, but you can't prevent it."

In other words, when you are selling sensible eating, do not pretend it will work miracles. It will not stop a whitehead from swelling ten minutes before a heavy date. It will not change basic shape; if you are big-boned, broad-hipped, short in the neck, the arm, or the leg, you will have to live with it, although at sixteen it may seem a ghastly fate. The advantage of sensible eating is that it helps you keep the best of what you have.

My theory, as you know, is to get the offspring when they are young and brainwash them in their preteens, before they ask too many questions. The next step, if you see by their build that they will have to be careful, is to read the riot act at puberty. This, again, is preventive medicine. Should older teens start to spread, despite your consistent efforts, the ideal is to move in firmly, gently, at the eight-pound excess level, when cutting down on a few sugars and starches should do the trick—if they will listen to you. (Try slipping them basic literature on diet and nutrition, which everyone should learn about anyhow.) When they are twenty pounds over, it is much harder to knock the weight off, but it can be done, especially by making the diet plan an integral part of normal family fare.

Young people do care how they look; they care desperately, even if they are genius level in math. They do not enjoy being fat. As for the maddening teen who consumes an outrageous amount of food, but looks healthy and does not gain a pound, let him alone. There may be some cryptic method to his eating, and bear in mind that a still-growing teen-ager needs more calories than an adult.

9

*Wheat Germ
or Garbage Bombs?*

According to its advocates, health food is salvation from body pollution; it makes you feel better and look better. Not so, its detractors claim. Health food is a rip-off, a colossal bore, and in itself no guarantee of good nutrition.

I do not pretend to know who is right. Certainly you can get fat from health food, as from anything else, if you eat too much of it. An excess of whole-grained breads, cakes, cookies, and snacks leads to fat just as quickly as too many pop-tarts or too much of Mom's apple pie.

No one ever mentions this, perhaps because most people who are tuned into health food do try to watch their weight —obesity is alien to their concept of well-being. This is particularly true of the young people in the movement for whom the old notion of being "fat and forty" seems like a form of depravity. The attitude holds, if less firmly, as adherents reach middle age, but, though it may be the fault of their previous habits, the rank and file of health food converts have never been noted for their vibrant good looks.

"I've taken vitamins and a quarter of a grain of thyroid for years now," says Diana Vreeland. "I eat lean instinctively, but I'm not health food–oriented. I see people in health food stores and they look like hell."

Perennial British TV star Katie Boyle, a rather stunning forty-two, fasts every Sunday on hot water, lemon, and honey to counteract compulsive eating but is not attracted by naturopathic diets. "A friend of mine," she once remarked in an interview, "came back from some huge health food conference and said, 'My dear, their bowels may be beautiful, but you should see their faces!'"

I am the first to regret that health food and the body beautiful are not an automatic equation. If they were, sunflower seeds would be sprouting out of my ears. I would even eat kelp. When you go to a beauty farm, particularly one of vegetarian persuasion, the gospel of organic, natural foods is rubbed into you with every massage. You come out slimmer, and the danger is in associating the two as cause and effect, conveniently forgetting how severely you were rationed.

To stay thin, you must learn to limit and balance your intake of food—the fact that it is unrefined, unsulfured, unadulterated, or cold-pressed does not change the issue. A yogurt a day, whether plain or laced with wheat germ, yeast, and honey, is excellent for you if you like it, but, of course, it contains calories. You do not just add it to your usual fare, you substitute it for some less nutritious item. Vitamin pills, however touted, often put an edge on appetite. If you notice this and feel reasonably sure that the food you eat provides enough vitamins, try cutting back on the pills. If not, and the swallowing soothes, go ahead.

"I take vitamins three times a day along with half a gram of thyroid," says columnist Suzy. "My impression is that I don't have nearly as many colds, but that is not why I started. The way I look at it is that, God knows, I need all the help I can get."

Betsy Bloomingdale, Arlene Dahl, and Janet Leigh also do their vitamin A, B, C, and E's. I conscientiously stoke up on a Swiss multi-vitamin, mineral, and ginseng compound every spring and fall, then let it slide unless I feel tired. Françoise de la Renta swears instead by protein tablets: "You take six a day. They give them to horses, and they're fantastic for the hair and skin. In the summer, you stop for two months to avoid becoming overaccustomed. Then you start again."

Food purist Merle Oberon puts both protein powder and vitamins in her yogurt and has replaced coffee with herbal teas. She infuses eucalyptus leaves when she has a cold, inhales the steam from the pot, and then drinks the strained brew. For those nasty liver spots on the hands, she recommends squeezing lemon juice on mother of pearl, which then corrodes. The following day, the resulting cream is spread on the spots to remove them. (Another technique, for what it is worth, is to pierce gelatin capsules of Vitamin E and smear the liquid on the back of the hands.)

Robin Hambro, wife of the English merchant banker, is another addict of both yogurt and herbal teas—in fact, of herbs in general. "In England, if your skin goes off, you can't sleep, or you just feel dreadful, you go to a homeopath or an aromatotherapist. If you have stomach trouble, they are liable to give you something to put in your bath. You try it and discover that it calms your stomach."

Checking this out with Madeleine Arcier, a London aromatotherapist, I found that customers indeed resort to massage with essential oils for a multitude of ills, including overweight. Aromatics are not health foods—you neither drink nor eat them. Nonetheless, through the use of pressure on points on the body, their locations derived mostly from Chinese acupuncture, the essences are thought to be absorbed through the skin to the greater therapeutic good. A special formula is worked out for each customer, and many of these contain oils from such common edibles as basil, rosemary, cinnamon, and sage.

Actress Elke Anderson goes farther afield for her favorite herbal pickups. She relies on African *piripiri,* the hottest pepper (grind together 25 percent piripiri and 75 percent gros sel and massage mixture into a flattened chicken prior to broiling). When tensions mount, she unwraps her Chinese ginseng root, takes a chew, or makes a tea from it. Her real idea of health food, however, is to go fishing (catch fish, slit open gullet, clean with sun and seawater, pop into boiling oil, and eat). Hopefully, I might add, the water is not polluted.

To be sure of prime quality, Cristina Ford, when home in Grosse Pointe, has an Italian grocer come every day at 8 A.M. with fruit and vegetables in season. She tries to have anything not indigenous flown in at its freshest and counts on a health food store for brown bread. She once drove over to a local farm to get free-range chickens, plopped them in the back of the car, and was horrified to discover they could not survive the trip. "You can imagine the mess in the Continental." Her solution was to build a chicken coop in a corner of the grounds where she could keep a few hens to give her fresh eggs.

At the same time, Cristina feels that if you really want to recharge the batteries, you have to take a vacation in some unspoiled place and forget daily precautions.

"It depends where," she adds. "I slipped off to Antigua to swim and eat the mangos right off the trees. But you don't live on mangos alone, and I also expected to find fresh fish. Instead, what I got was U.S. frozen. How lazy people are! I waved it away—unless you do, you'll never see anything fresh again."

But even when it is fresh, how do you know it is safe? Stubbornly, I continue to insist on as much fresh produce in season as I can find—I happen to care about flavor—but suspicion of declining integrity nags. We are all becoming slightly paranoid about food: another reason it amazes me that anyone would want to eat too much. I do not think that restricting yourself to "official" health foods is either possible or desirable; they cost too much even for my household, and in some cases they are dreary, or not as pure as they purport to be. While I am fond of brown rice, for example, whole-grained pasta is a disaster.

Needless to say, when in New York, where health food stores abound, I am the first to slip in and buy whatever might give me a boost. It is like buying insurance—after all, you never know. Back in Rome, I do not bother. Romans are not yet preoccupied with health food, and specialized stores are two in number (for three million inhabitants). On the one hand, it seems that everything from cheese, oil, wine to water has been doctored for the worse. More than adultery, Italy is the land of adulteration. On the other hand, though I hate to think what is done to our fruit and vegetables, our imported meat, or the few Italian chickens made to scratch for their supper, they all still have a distinctive taste. There have been investigations of possibly cancerous baking techniques, yet the thick Italian loaves still seem wholesome. Are we living on borrowed time before we too succumb to processed paradise? I hope not.

Baroness Pauline de Rothschild says she has not touched a mussel since she saw the polluted state of certain famous mussel beds. I, for one, with great regret, have written off almost all Italian shellfish. Friends of mine still eat it, but they make the sign of the horns to ward off typhoid and hepatitis. It is the loss of quality in food that is the saddest, both for health and aesthetics—no longer to be able to order a supreme diet lunch of two dozen oysters and a dry white wine without questioning the validity of either.

The horror of instant refueling has long been apparent.

The baroness also recalls her instinctive withdrawal from a toasted-cheese sandwich she ordered in the Paris airport when rushing to catch a plane. She did not expect it would taste like Croque Monsieur, that more leisurely version of the same snack. What struck her was that the counterboy, surely following instructions, heated the dreary thing still wrapped in tinfoil. Was that supposed to enrich the bread?

Easy as it is to scoff at such health foods as powdered yeast and nut cutlets, it is clear that they or, for that matter, the less drastic forms of macrobiotics, can be more palatable than highly processed foods. Mimi Sheraton, in an article for *New York* magazine, quotes Harvard's Dr. Jean Mayer, former presidential adviser on nutrition: "Some commercial soft drink labels read like a qualitative analysis of the East River. . . . The less the number of additives we can get away with, the better." She adds that the current number is about three thousand, plus some fifteen hundred artificial flavorings.

Rightly or wrongly, after the DDT, mercury, MSG, and cyclamates scares, it seems foolish to gamble that other extraneous gunk in modern food is harmless. Mind you, if the wonder concentrates, ready-mades, and TV frozens tasted divine, I might not be adverse to them. But whether or not the additives are dangerous, the non-flavor of convenience foods is enough to put me off. Recently there has been an onslaught of consumer protection articles urging the housewife to decipher the fine print on labels regarding ingredients as well as net weights. In other words, she should comparison shop among the welter of packages for the best nutrition as well as a bargain price. Even to a speed-reader, it must be apparent that broiling a slice of liver is less time-consuming than reading all those labels, and furthermore, how do you evaluate seventy-one kinds of potato chips and a gondola full of non-dairy toppings? My advice is to ignore them—save your eyes and your tastebuds for greater pleasures.

As for your figure, one theory holds that, if you are fat, you should avoid processed foods above all else because the emulsifiers and additives they contain form what are known as long chains. While the food industry claims that you eliminate emulsifiers, it is quite possible that they continue to function in the body as inert or still collectors. In simple terms, this means that they "make fat." In addition, most vitamins are removed from processed foods because vitamins make food spoilable. No wonder bottles of multi-vitamin pills sit on the American table next to the salt and pepper.

"If I were a mold, I would take exception to U.S. bread," says Dr. Mark D. Altschule. "I couldn't live on it; very few beings can. In order to have frozen or canned food that keeps, you have to take out so much that even the weevils sneer. Many years ago, about half the patients in this country's mental hospitals were there because of vitamin deficiencies resulting from malnutrition. Ironically, this has been pretty well wiped out among the lower classes, but it still exists in the upper classes—the lower classes may have to buy cheap meat and cheap vegetables, but at least they can't afford frozen and other convenience food. Thank God a lot of middle-class kids in America still grow up where they can dig worms—if the soil is rich enough to contain them, worms are nutritious."

In the light of this and other statements from concerned professionals, Adelle Davis recipes begin to sound gourmet (her ideas have always been fascinating), and one dismisses less blithely the rumblings and fulminations of the cultists. Extremist attitudes do not appeal to me, but are rolled oats and soy sauce any more extreme than a diet based on fatburgers, fat dogs, and assorted sugars?

Russell Baker, in one of his brilliant columns for *The New York Times,* hit upon the notion of the garbage bomb as the ultimate capitalist weapon. In his opinion the only sensible way to think of any modern war is to view it as a garbagedisposal system. In other words, load the B-52's with beer cans, plastic bottles, and aerosol cans and "start dumping thirty-ton loads of frozen TV dinners that nobody back home could stand to eat." Naturally, Mr. Baker also had other forms of contemporary garbage in mind—not just edibles and their lethal containers. But what a splendid solution! Put the agribusiness overflow, which is no good to us, into the service of defense, take the most tasteless, ersatz items off the shelves, and put them into the stockpile of armaments that will keep the world safe for democracy. For a start, just our A-for-airline and H-for-hospital food would give us fantastic overkill in the G-bomb department. The list of other ready-mades is endless—if we stored them in arsenals now and threw away the keys, we would be both leaner and stronger overnight.

10

Men Who Measure Up

Kikuyu Chief Nijiiri, the ruler of three thousand acres on the slopes of Mount Kenya, has outlived thirty of his fifty-four wives. He has fathered more than 185 children—the exact total is unknown because years ago he stopped counting them. At age 111, his powers somewhat diminished, he wraps his imposing frame in monkey skins when supervising the work of his remaining wives on the land.

In an article for *The Sunday Times* of London, Henry Reuter quoted him as follows: "When you have as many wives as I have had, you have to be a diplomat. For many, many years I called three of them every night. I wanted as many children as possible, and God was good to me—I helped him a little by eating such foods as milk, meat, and honey, with an occasional mashed sweet potato, very good for keeping a man strong."

On the other hand, Dr. Joseph B. Trainer, associate professor of physiology at the University of Oregon Medical School, has described the average American male as a disaster. "He eats too much. He sits in front of the tube with a glass of beer. He goes to sleep on the sofa. Finally, he wakes up enough to go to bed—and to sleep." The professor further blasts the U.S. male as "overweight, over-tobaccoed, over-alcoholed, and under-sexed."

Maybe the problem is lack of wives? Could it be lack of land? I prefer to think, since I married one, that the American male is not to be scrapped. I cannot vouch for what happens at 111, but at forty-nine he holds his own.

Admittedly, the most attractive men over thirty watch what they eat and drink—just like the chief. The first thing they cut is carbohydrates, which makes sense by all modern reckoning. They cut but do not necessarily eliminate them altogether, which could be a smart idea—who knows what power lies in the heart of a sweet potato? I confess the idea haunts me.

Men who stay in shape also exercise. Once you graduate from the playing fields, city-suburban existence is sedentary all the way. Unless you play sports or work out regularly, within ten years the brawn goes to pot. You wind up like Elizabeth Taylor protesting to grips on location who teased for her for overeating: "That's not fat, that's muscle." Thrust it up, suck it in, fat is fat, and you will never have that Taylor beauty as compensation.

"My weight didn't change much for years," says outdoorsman, writer-producer Peter Gimbel. "Before thirty-four, I felt I could eat anything. Then I went on the expedition to shoot *Blue Water, White Death.* For long periods, we were short of food. Whenever we got where we could eat, we gorged. Back home in New York, I used to window-shop pastry shops and delicatessens. One day I got on the scale and saw that number 200 approach. I was appalled. I'm tall enough so that twenty pounds wasn't that obvious, but I'd rather be five pounds under than over. Fat disgusts me.

"I went to a doctor for a checkup and told him about this weird compulsion. His reaction was: 'Very interesting.' He had had concentration camp survivors with subsequent over-weight problems. The psychological trauma had been too fierce—they couldn't pass up food.

"With me it was temporary. I weigh about 175 now, which is what I weighed twenty years ago. I'm conscious of not eating stuff that's fattening. You have to be. Sometimes I pass up something I'd really like, but mostly it's enough to avoid bread, potatoes, desserts, and to eat only when I'm hungry. I drink, but I don't nibble on the cocktail garbage—if any-thing, a carrot stick. I have an iron gut; I don't get sick, and although I'm very concerned about ecology, I'm absolutely unconcerned about 'eating pollution.' In fact, I almost try to contaminate myself—my dog who sniffs in the gutter gives me a kiss in the morning. I do take vitamins: a once-a-day broad-spectrum pill and 2,000 mg of vitamin C—my 'rolfer' talked me into it.

"Rolfing," he continues, "is a massage technique named after Ida Rolf, who developed it years ago. She believed that the physical aging process starts in the connective tissue, in-cluding the fasciae, which become nonlubricated, wrinkled, and damaged. As stress builds up because of physical or emo-tional tension, the muscles don't slide as they should. I had a bad back for fifteen years, nothing that could be diagnosed; after ten rolfing sessions of an hour and a half each, it was cured. The technique is rough—when my rolfer found a knot in the back of the thigh, he would place his elbow there and put his whole weight against it.

"I don't do calisthenics. For me, they're bad karma, though I would love to be a fly on the wall in a gym; most of the men there look so absurd. The way I see it, rolfing is a kind of instant yoga. After rolfing, I thought it over and came to the conclusion that aging is tension and the answer for me was yoga. It's the most marvelous system I've ever seen for the body, and it's mind-boggling as well."

I must say, though I find it simpler and more effective to stay in shape by doing calisthenics, I'm beginning to have second thoughts—those yoga people look so marvelous. Maybe it works best for men; not that it necessarily should. I gather from Rome yogi Grant Muradoff that in true yoga men must do the women's movements and vice versa. The fact that, to varying degrees, we are all both male and female, is what brings the balance. I suspect life would be easier were we not, but we are.

"If you exercise you feel better; I do yoga," Frecky Vreeland says. "I was president of the Yoga Society of Morocco. It's more than exercise, it's a way of life that gets you going in the right direction. The greatest luxury is to have a place in the bedroom or bathroom to do a few positions at the drop of a hat without having to push things aside or pull down the curtains and worry about privacy. If you do only one thing, you should do the shoulder stand to reverse circulation.

"Sleep, too, is important, and everything else is food. I do believe one is what one eats. You try to find out what the healthy foods are, eliminating the others. It's so simple to say, 'Give me two vegetables and no potatoes.' Obviously, if someone who's with you has French fries, you reach over and eat as many as you can get away with. If you can limit drinking to wine, it's infinitely better than the rest of the stuff—not that I can do it. As far as the stimulation is concerned, one's 'button clicking' adjusts to whatever one's drinking. It used to be that it took one-and-a-half martinis for the button to click. Instead of escalating, I deescalated, and now I find that a half jigger of whiskey or vodka will do it. The people who've had two dry martinis all their life before every meal are the ones who show it."

Frecky's son Nicholas, a student at the American College in Paris who has been working with photographer Irving Penn during summer vacations, is even leaner than his father. He takes it for granted—the least one might expect at that age.

"I don't even bother to eat reasonably," he says, "and I've got this crazy grandmother who already tells me: 'Oh, Nicky, you must do exercises in front of the mirror.' " If he ever needs to, he will. With his background, he cannot afford to be fat.

One of my favorite designers, Giorgio Sant'Angelo, is also into yoga and organics and has a very special eating regime I personally would not recommend, though it seems to work beautifully for him.

"I'm five feet eight, I weigh 125 and have for twenty years or more," he explains. "I swim as much as I can—I have an indoor pool in the country—and when I can't swim, I do yoga or go into my pillow. In any movement, it's terribly important that your mind or a certain happiness be involved; that's why most exercise is a waste of time. Stretching, as in yoga, makes you feel wonderful and keeps you resilient."

"Did you say pillow?"

"Yes, my pillow has made all the difference. Really it's a big pillowcase I made out of stretch fabric lined with cotton—synthetics are unpleasant to the skin—with holes for the arms and head. I'm the stuffing, only I don't stay still. Once inside, I let the spirit move me. I loll, roll around, curl up, extend a knee, or kick against the sides. It's like pushing against a stream of water. You have no idea what marvelous shapes the pillow acquires."

I can imagine. In fact, for those days when everything goes wrong, I can think of nothing better than having a few pillows around the house to climb into for a collective revel on the floor. Furthermore, it is too bad one dresses for a party because the pillow could be the icebreaker of all time.

"I have an uncle in Switzerland who's a dietician," Giorgio continues. "I was brought up to eat very little. I never eat during the day: only liquids or, if I need something, boiled vegetables. I never have business lunches. At night, I often have two dinners, one when I get home and another if I go out. I'm a night person. I have chicken or fish—red meat takes me three days to digest—but otherwise at night I eat whatever I want. I drink only wine; I don't take vitamins. I get a minimum of eight hours sleep, keep a low metabolism, and really have no problems."

Businessmen Bernard Lanvin and Yves Vidal adhere instead to a more conventional pattern: anti-carbohydrate, pro-calisthenics. Both of them have gyms set up at home. They follow no rigid diet routine, nor are they concerned with health food supplements.

"It's true that when I'm in Morocco, my life is healthier and the fish, vegetables, and fruit seem fresher," says Yves, whose ancient fortress-castle dominates Tangiers. "I never know what my cook will bring back from the market. If I suggest sole, I'm liable to find *rougets* for lunch. The cook will explain that she couldn't buy sole because they were dead. If the fish doesn't jump in her basket, she won't buy.

"I don't expect this in Paris, nor do I try to duplicate the same food conditions. Quite simply, I pay attention to what I eat. You try to use your intelligence with food as with everything else. It's a question of equilibrium and self-control. I'm a no-breakfast man except for tea with lemon—never sugar, which I hate. I don't even drink coffee with sugar; if when I'm out I'm passed a cup with sugar in the bottom, I can't drink it, so obviously, I don't like cakes and pastry. I avoid carbohydrates in general, which means I don't eat bread and potatoes. It just so happens I like green vegetables better. If I feel like it, I have spaghetti in Italy, and I certainly am not adverse to cassoulet [roughly, pork and beans], but it's the exception, not the rule. I tend to drink very little; the real secret is never touch liquor after dinner—you continue instead with wine or champagne.

"Eating sensibly is much better than any fat farm or crash diet. I don't believe in calorie counting. It's impossible, a terrible bore, and you wind up in a foul temper. And basically, being thin isn't what counts—it's not letting yourself go. I have a gym set up at home. I work out three times a week with an instructor, usually at lunchtime. Then I eat a *grillade,* which takes me about five minutes." Yves, who is forty-nine and six feet tall, has weighed about 158 pounds since the end of World War II.

Bernard Lanvin, at thirty-six, belongs to a younger generation. Six feet, two inches tall, he weighs about 167 pounds.

"My weight isn't distributed exactly the way I'd like it; there could be less around the waist," Lanvin says. Attired in a dapper pinstripe suit, he looked fine to me—not a hint of paunch, and I do not think it was only the tailoring.

"I don't watch what I eat all that much," he adds, "though I do weigh myself every morning. I've put on ten pounds since I've been married, and I'm only too aware, in my business, that the average Frenchman grows a belly. Either he tends to by constitution or he just doesn't bother to take care of himself. Once past thirty-five, you cut down on butter, eat less bread, and drink less wine (especially at lunch)—I don't like apéritifs and booze, but I do like a good red wine with dinner. No, I don't take vitamins!

"When I can, I stop off at the Automobile Club on my way home to swim a few lengths of the pool. Weekends, I golf or play tennis. In the winter I try to slip off and ski. Come what may, excluding business trips, I start my day three times a week at 7:30 A.M. with a brisk workout at home. It seems I grew up doing calisthenics, and if you stop, you find that your mental/physical balance goes off. In a way, it's a question of organization—to keep your professional and family life going and still find time for sports, you have to get organized. As far as fat is concerned, I'm probably lucky; I'm just not built to put on weight—not that I don't suck in my stomach like everyone else when I go to the beach."

Parisian writer-socialite José Luis de Villalonga's advice from the more difficult graying-at-the-temples stage of life is both sensible and drastic. Its main merit is that it works for him. In other words he, like every mature man, has had to come to some personal reckoning: if you want to present a certain image to the world, you make an effort to preserve it. His formula runs roughly as follows: no dieting, but at the same time no bread, butter, pastry, or liquor—the latter is death. Once a week take a mild sleeping pill and go to bed at seven o'clock. There is nothing like twelve to eighteen hours sleep to recharge the batteries. Have a good massage from time to time to aid circulation. Get as much fresh air and sun as possible and avoid nightclubs: "They're as bad as cancer."

"Above all," he says, "avoid boring people; they put wrinkles on the soul. A tedious dinner party can age you two years."

Having sat through many, I heartily agree, although when I had to endure such dinners in quantity, I was young enough to shrug them off. I also agree that for both men and women some highly individual form of regular discipline is the best answer.

Skipping meals will not do. The average Roman businessman, caught in the one o'clock traffic on his way home to lunch, has a nervous breakdown. Once home, should the pasta not be cooked, there are further hysterics. Less pasta and more breakfast might help.

Diuretics and slimming pills are also a disaster, particularly for intense, active men. For the temporary loss of a few pounds, you and everyone around you start climbing the walls. I remember Count Luciano della Porta rushing off from sun and surf at Copacabana Beach to cable his diet doctor. He could not remember what color pill to take at noon, and he was in a panic at the thought of possibly taking the wrong one. Another once-relevant case is that of the brilliant film director Roberto Rossellini.

"It's not true that Roberto doesn't care about his weight. He cares, but usually he doesn't do anything. He likes to eat," his cousin Franco explained. "So he tried these pills. He wasn't hungry; they made him angry instead. It got so the family hid them or fled the house whenever he was there. What's the point of being slender and sensational if the way you do it makes you totally neurotic?"

With men, as with women, there is little doubt that build as well as discipline counts. It is not fair (or scientifically proved), but even as far as weight is concerned, some people seem to be more equal than others. All the more credit, for example, to the Gianni Bulgaris of this world. He, like me, would be gross in a year if he did not keep a falcon (preferably Byzantine and jeweled) on his shoulder, an imaginary falcon to swoop down on prey he has to leave on his plate. Both he and I suffered fat in early adolescence—enough to put us on guard for life. When it comes to the pleasure of food, however sensual, there is no choice: we have to be voyeurs. Nor are we alone.

"There were two guys," Van Johnson says, "who always ate like truck drivers: Bob Taylor and Jimmy Stewart. I finally decided their glands are balanced and mine aren't. At six feet three, age fifty-six, I'd settle for 205 pounds, but I'll never see that again. I love beer, I love wine. I love champagne and double vodkas on the rocks. Five years ago, while doing a picture, a lady hypnotist got hold of me. I was so hung up on smoking, I could have two Salems and three Tampax lit at the same time. Five minutes with her, and smoking was over. The only trouble was I went right into food. I've got to find that broad again to see what she can do about eating.

"I'm a big disciple of high protein, though I know all that meat and water must be ripping the kidneys. I can just see where it leads: dribbling all night with the wastebasket close by the bed in a hotel room. I'm also a banana junkie (that's potassium)—whenever you're hungry, have a glass of skimmed milk and grab a banana, but there's a limit, or else you turn into an ape. Vitamins? Jesus, yes! Three C's, three E's, and all the others, including double B_{12} shots when I'm on the road. I also believe in honey.

"The problem is that in between jobs I nosh. I plant the

tulips, hyacinths, and daffodils, and I go to the icebox. At the moment, I've tapered off—I've put a picture of Audrey Hepburn, all bones and hollows, on the fridge so that I get there and say, 'OK, Audrey,' and crawl away."

Van Johnson exaggerates. We all know he looks divine and always will. Quite simply, he knows himself physically, as any actor must, or for that matter, as any person must if he wants to stay in shape. Most beautiful people are so conditioned (and perhaps so constructed) that they never put on more than five pounds. Van Johnson, like Princess Ira Furstenberg, has to put up more of a fight. Ira, not trusting herself on her own, slips into a clinic the minute her weight goes up; Van Johnson has the sense of humor to see him through the direst of fat farm restrictions. If splurge and repent, neglect and clean house, gives you better balance than walking a daily tightrope, by all means play it that way. It is the result that counts.

Balance your diet or, if you prefer, consciously unbalance it, as long as you are aware of yourself and the orthodox rules. Do your push-ups or yoga asanas; have your wheat germ, vitamins, yeast; eat food when it is fresh; boycott the ersatz; pull in that stomach, tuck in that bottom: it is up to you to find what keeps you happily lean. Splurge without regret, but only when the splurging is truly superb. Basically, you as well as I know what to do day by day, month by month, and no one has to tell us. All the diet books in the world can be summed up in four words: eat little and exercise.